TACKLING CHILD OBESITY WITH HENRY

HEALTH EXERCISE NUTRITION FOR THE REALLY YOUNG

A handbook for community and health practitioners

Candida Hunt & Mary Rudolf

ACKNOWLEDGEMENTS

We are grateful to our colleagues who contributed to the development of this book:

Professor Jane Barlow, University of Warwick
Professor Sarah Cowley, Kings College London
Professor Hilton Davis, Kings College London
Dr Penny Gibson, Advisor on Obesity, RCPCH
Professor Neil McIntosh, RCPCH Vice-President
Dr Lisa Mohebati
Bernadette Mulley, Specialist Health Visitor, Leeds PCT
Dr Pinki Sahota, Leeds Metropolitan University
Professor Carolyn Summerbell, University of Teesside

We would also like to thank Jan Burkhardt, Dr Deborah Christie, Dr Laurel Edmunds, Sue Hanson, the Family Links Nurturing Programme, the University of Warwick's Families for Health programme and the WATCH IT programme, whose ideas and approaches have influenced the development of HENRY. Thanks too to the Glugs team for the HENRY toolkit.

HENRY was originally developed with funding from the Child Growth Foundation and then from the Department of Health and the Department for Children, Schools and Families, and with the support of the Royal College of Paediatrics and Child Health.

www.henry.org.uk

First published in the UK in 2008 by
Unite/Community Practitioners' and Health Visitors' Association
Tel: 0207 505 3000 Fax: 0207 780 4142
www.unitetheunion.com

ISBN: 978-1-872278-74-2

£10.00 Members
£12.00 Non-members

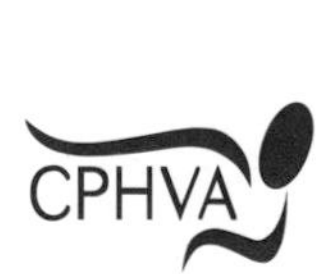

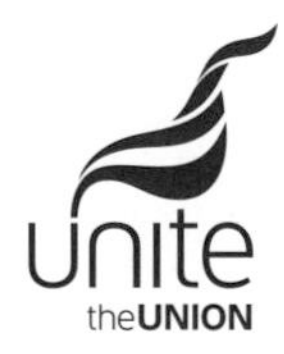

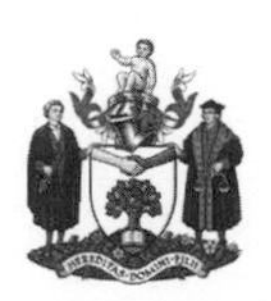

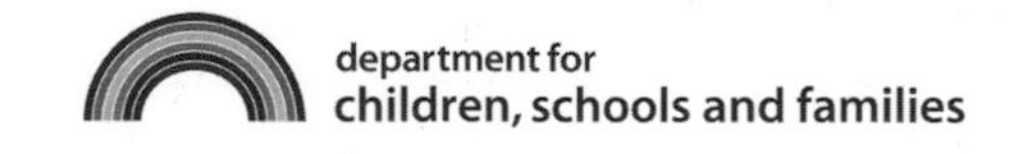

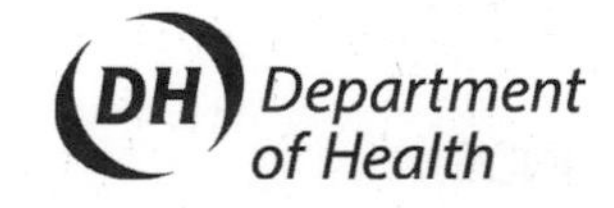

CONTENTS

PART ONE

PART TWO

PART THREE

FOREWORD

I am delighted to contribute a Foreword to this timely and informative book on the HENRY approach.

As National Clinical Director for Children at the Department of Health, I have observed the overwhelming evidence of the emerging obesity epidemic, which threatens the health, duration and quality of life of future generations.

The Foresight Project *Tackling Obesities: Future Choices* (2007) was a wake-up call for us all, and the government has responded by publishing *Healthy Weight: Healthy Lives* (2008). However, policy developments alone will not suffice. We need the children's workforce, especially in the early years, to be fully engaged in supporting families right from the start.

The problems of childhood obesity are not proving easy to tackle. However, there is new information. It is important to continue research and also to ensure that the evidence base is translated into practical approaches, which this book sets out to achieve. Both preventing and also reversing obesity is imperative for the UK, and is now a global concern.

Our new *Child Health Promotion Programme* aims to ensure that every baby has the opportunity to become a healthy child. Breastfeeding initiation and continuation is key. We need to do more to support mothers, and to involve fathers too. Weaning is a critical stage. How children eat, as well as what they eat, matters – and we must refocus on activity levels too.

Much of this field raises new concerns for practitioners, who want more information on the correct approach.

I know this book will be warmly welcomed and widely read. It is an invaluable guide with a modern, evidence-based approach, enabling parents to receive the best support available today from well-informed and skilful practitioners.

Sheila Shribman

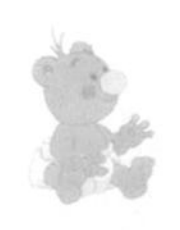

ABOUT THIS BOOK

Levels of obesity are rising so fast in children today that the issue has been described as a time bomb. Only a few years ago the problem was limited to teenagers, but the age when obesity begins to affect children has been decreasing, and now as many as 10% of children are obese as they start school. The latest research has shown that preschoolers and even babies are affected. As a result childhood obesity is now a key issue on the national agenda, and the government has set targets to reduce levels of obesity in children as they start school.

Tackling childhood obesity through focusing on the early years is central to the new national Child Health Promotion Programme. Community and health practitioners working with young families need to be in the front line in attempts to prevent the development of obesity. You have expertise in advising and supporting families, and may be the first port of call for parents with concerns. Unfortunately, our research both with parents of young obese children and with health practitioners has shown that there is a serious lack of confidence and skills in working with parents and carers on this issue. Because the epidemic has only recently affected this young age group, there has been little training available to provide practitioners with an effective approach for helping young children at risk of obesity.

We developed HENRY – Health Exercise Nutrition for the Really Young – to give practitioners the knowledge and the practical skills you need to influence parents and help them provide a home environment that will most benefit their children. The HENRY approach is underpinned by current evidence relating to obesity, parenting and lifestyle, and adopts the Family Partnership Model, a way of working proven to be of benefit in supporting parents. It involves reflective practice, and takes a strengths-based approach to helping families find their own solutions and the motivation to put these into practice. In 2007 HENRY was funded by the Department of Health and the Department for Children, Schools and Families. Training courses have been successfully piloted, and are now available nationwide. HENRY is cited in key government documents such as the *Child Health Promotion Programme* and *Healthy Weight, Healthy Lives Guidance*.

Tackling Child Obesity with HENRY explores the theory, the evidence base and the practical context for our work, and offers ideas and resources to use with parents. It is designed both as a stand-alone resource and as background reading for HENRY training courses. (See www.henry.org.uk for more information.) We hope that the book will prove of value to community and health practitioners who take up the challenge of helping parents provide their children with an optimally healthy start to life.

Candida Hunt & Mary Rudolf

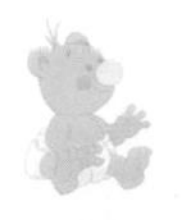

BACKGROUND

PART ONE

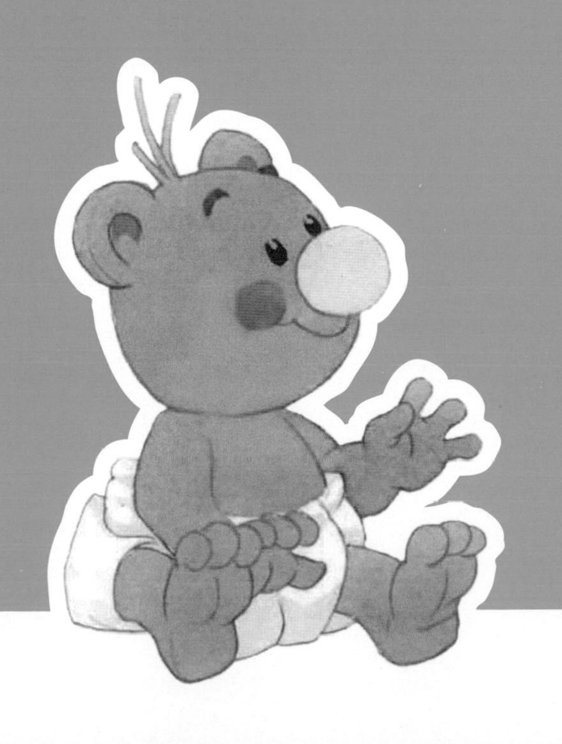

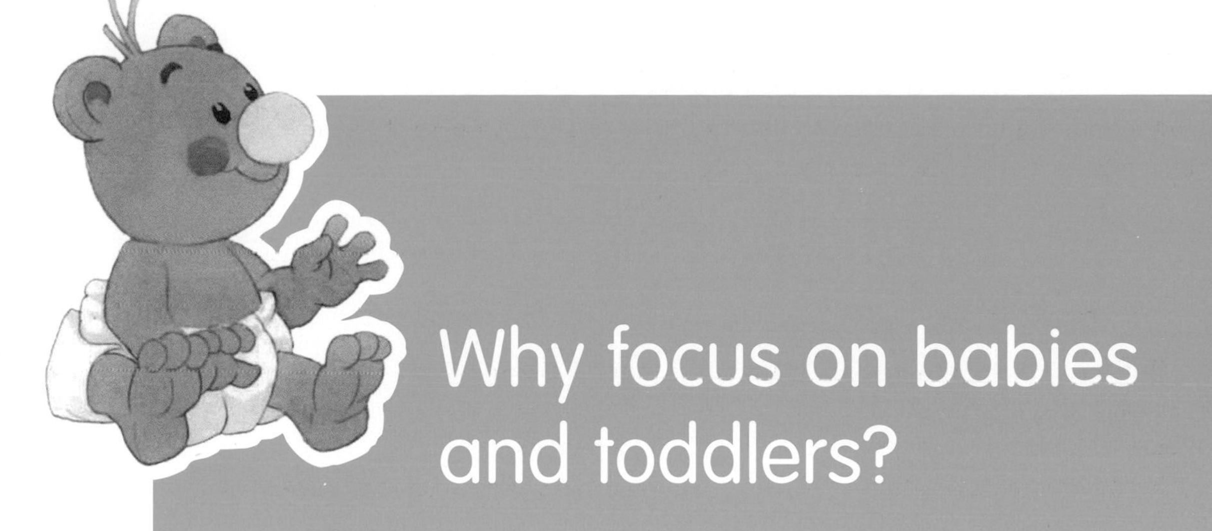

Why focus on babies and toddlers?

Most societies see a 'bonny' baby as being desirable, and weight gain as an indicator of health and well-being. Only rarely are parents concerned when their baby is chubby, and if they are, the traditional professional response has been reassurance that fat babies slim down once they start walking.

Should we be changing our attitudes? The answer is undoubtedly yes. Evidence from around the world is accumulating that both rapid weight gain and obesity in the early months – even the first weeks – of life are linked to the development of long-term obesity. The risks are so considerable that obese infants are up to ten times more likely to become obese later than thinner babies are. Some studies have even directly linked obesity in infancy to obesity in adult life.

There is even stronger evidence that obesity in childhood tracks into adult life. We know that being obese as a child carries a number of health risks in childhood as well as beyond. So, although we do not yet have evidence that intervening in the early years can improve one's health in later life, it is logical to assume that it is likely to be helpful. In fact the argument that we should be targeting the very young becomes more powerful when we consider that one primary school child in three in the UK is already overweight and one in five is obese, so a very large proportion of children are heading towards obesity whatever their growth pattern in infancy.

Why does obesity in childhood matter so much?

It is worth summarising the range of health problems that obese children may develop during their school years. In the table below, problems that present for medical attention are shown on the left, but of greater concern are the hidden problems shown on the right, which are found only if one looks for them. These are alarmingly common – research

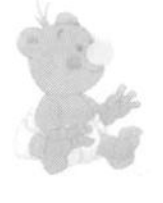

studies from the United States show that as many as 58% of obese children have one of these problems and 25% have two or more.

HEALTH PROBLEMS AFFECTING OBESE CHILDREN

Overt problems	Problems that may be concealed
Emotional and behavioural difficulties	The metabolic syndrome
Asthma	Polycystic ovary syndrome
Sleep disorders	Hypertension
Orthopaedic complications	Non-alcoholic fatty liver disease
Skin problems	Impaired glucose tolerance
Gall bladder disease	
Pseudotumour cerebri	
Type 2 diabetes	

This knowledge offers the most powerful reason why we should intervene in childhood. If obese children can develop metabolic problems such as glucose intolerance, diabetes, high cholesterol and high blood pressure even before they reach puberty, then we should be attempting to prevent these problems early. This is especially true if their parents are obese or have diabetes, as their risks are then even higher.

Should we wait until later in childhood to intervene? The answer is almost definitely no. Obesity in very young children is not necessarily benign. Some severely obese toddlers and young children suffer from sleep apnoea and orthopaedic problems. More worrying is the finding that early signs of atherosclerosis are already present in obese children as young as 3–8 years old. Perhaps the strongest reason is an optimism that it may be easier to prevent or reverse obesity early in life when children are most impressionable and lifestyle patterns are yet to be established.

Why are we seeing an increase in obesity now?

Genes and the environment act together to make an individual susceptible to obesity, and it is often difficult to disentangle which is at play. On a population level, the recent upsurge in obesity can only be explained by factors in the environment, as genes can hardly have changed in the last decade or so. Intrauterine factors also seem to have a role. Babies who are born large are more likely to be obese, as are babies whose mothers are obese during pregnancy. This is concerning as it suggests that some obesity may be programmed during foetal life and so may be even harder to reverse.

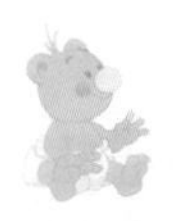

1

Environmental factors relate to nutrition, eating behaviour and physical activity, and it is easy to see that in recent years there has been a massive change in lifestyle that could account for the epidemic we are facing. In order to begin to address these factors we need to explore the evidence. Are children consuming inappropriate foods that exceed their needs? Are children less active than they used to be and so need fewer calories than previously?

Specific questions of interest are:

- Does it matter if a baby is breast- or bottle-fed?
- Is weaning an important period?
- What do young children eat and is it of good quality?
- How do young children eat and what influences their pattern of eating?
- How active are children today and what influence does television have?

Breast or bottle?

A heated debate has been aired for some years about whether the way babies are fed has an influence on the development of obesity. There is now good evidence that breastfeeding is protective – the likelihood that a baby will become obese is reduced by as much as 20% to 45% if they are breast-fed. In-depth analysis of the research shows that this protection increases if breastfeeding is exclusive and if infants are breast-fed for longer. The lowest risk is for babies who breast feed for more than 6 months. This is important information as it provides further impetus to attempts to improve breastfeeding rates. Interestingly the protective effect is seen more in adolescence than it is in childhood.

A look at babies' growth charts emphasises that there is a difference between the growth of breast- and bottle-fed babies. The charts in current use are for the most part made up from information on the growth of formula-fed babies. New (World Health Organisation) charts are being introduced in the UK that have been derived from breast-fed babies, and they are different. By the time breast-fed babies are 12 months old, they are longer and lighter than formula-fed babies, and fewer of them are above the 91st centile for weight.

A number of explanations have been given for how breastfeeding might protect a baby from developing obesity. The first focuses on how we learn to regulate our energy intake. Breast-fed babies control their own intake of milk, and adjust it according to how satiated they feel. Bottle-fed babies, on the other hand, are provided with a quantity of milk which they may be encouraged to finish even when they are full. Over time, this difference may lead to a baby's natural self-regulation being overridden.

Support for this idea comes from research showing that there is a difference between breast- and bottle-fed babies at weaning. Formula-fed babies continue to take the same volume of milk as before, whereas breast-fed babies reduce their intake of milk, adjusting it for calories they are receiving from solid food. Another finding of interest relating to self-regulation is that babies who routinely finish the bottle are more likely to become obese than those who tend to leave some undrunk.

A further explanation for why breastfeeding is protective relates to metabolic programming early in life. Breast milk and formula milk are not the same, and babies' hormonal responses to milks differ. It has been shown that insulin levels are higher in formula-fed babies, and that they have a prolonged response to insulin by the time they are six days old. Insulin has a potent influence on growth in the first year of life, and higher levels stimulate greater fat deposition, with a link to obesity developing during childhood. Another hormone, leptin, has also been implicated. Leptin is a key regulator of appetite and body fatness. Animal studies show that breast milk contains leptin at the end of a feed, and it is thought that the leptin may signal to the suckling's brain that enough has been taken. Another study showed that when baby rats are overfed before they are weaned they tend to become overweight and resistant to leptin later in life.

When considering why breastfeeding tends to protect against obesity we need to bear in mind that there may be other factors contributing, about which we have less influence. Breastfeeding rates are known to be higher among mothers who are more educated, who may well have a better appreciation of the importance of nutrition. They are also likely to be more active. Some of the protective effects of breastfeeding may therefore be due to the baby being born into a healthier, less obesogenic family environment.

Apart from the protective effect against obesity, there is an additional benefit of breastfeeding that is less well recognised. Babies who are breast-fed are exposed to a wide variety of tastes that are denied a bottle-fed baby, as flavours of food eaten by the mother are transmitted through her milk. A baby offered these same foods at weaning accepts them more readily! This makes some sense biologically as it means that young mammals are programmed to be receptive to the taste of foods that their mother eats and are therefore likely to be safe. They are less receptive to those foods that she has avoided, which might be potentially harmful. A series of fascinating experiments has shown that babies exposed to carrots during pregnancy and lactation accept carrots more readily than formula-fed babies do (see Chapter 6). It has also been shown that the more varied a mother's diet is during pregnancy and lactation, the more likely it is that an infant will accept new flavours. Encouraging mothers to eat a healthy and varied diet could help to avoid the eating difficulties that are so common in young children today.

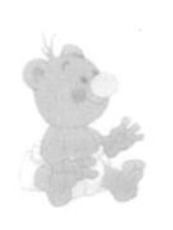

In summary, breastfeeding is protective against obesity, and brings a number of other benefits that optimise a baby's health. The message is clear – increasing the number of babies who are breast-fed for longer could have a considerable effect on the epidemic of obesity that we are trying to tackle.

Key ideas

- Promoting exclusive breastfeeding for longer periods is important
- Encouraging mothers to eat a variety of desired foods such as fruit and vegetables during pregnancy and lactation may lead to an improvement in their children's diets

The importance of the weaning period

The World Health Organisation's guidance that solid foods should only be introduced at six months is highly controversial. The major reason for the recommendation is to reduce risks of infection in developing countries, but there is good evidence that delaying weaning is also beneficial in reducing obesity.

The age when solids are started relates to the development of obesity: rates are higher in babies who have been weaned before they are 16 weeks old. So the timing of weaning is important, as is the sort of food introduced at weaning.

One of the biggest culprits is fruit juice – something not usually thought to be a weaning food. Babies are commonly given fruit juice in the very early weeks of life. It is not surprising, given our natural preference for sweet tastes, that many babies then refuse water and drink only juice. This habit may not cause excessive weight gain directly, but it does have a metabolic effect. Animal studies show that insulin levels rise and this, as we have already seen, can promote fat deposition.

The solid food given at weaning is often poor – excessively high in calories, and with inadequate amounts of fruit and vegetables. Studies from the United States show that the energy intake of American infants only 7–11 months old exceeds their requirements by as much as 20–30%, and that over the following year this rises further. The transition to table foods worsens the situation as it often involves high-calorie foods. We have no reason for confidence that British toddlers eat any better than American toddlers: UK surveys show that many rarely eat fruit and vegetables, and that most babies have sampled chocolate by the time they are 12 months old.

Weaning is therefore an important period when we could intervene with good effect. The importance of this goes beyond simply avoiding undesirable high-calorie foods that promote the development of fat. Recent research tells us that eating habits are established early in life and then track into childhood and adulthood, so children can be primed to eat more desirable foods. A good example that illustrates this is nutramigen, a special formula given to babies with gastrointestinal problems. This formula has a particularly unpleasant taste, and is rejected if it is not started very early in life before tastes are fully developed. Infants who have been fed this formula have been shown to have a heightened preference later on in childhood for tastes that have the flavour and aroma of nutramigen – broccoli is a notable example!

We need to work towards improving babies' diets at weaning, not only to ensure that these are healthy and not excessive in calories, but also to influence their likes and preferences, which may well have a lifelong influence on foods eaten later in life.

Key ideas

- Weaning influences an individual's programming for obesity
- It is optimal to delay the introduction of solid foods until 6 months
- Juice is undesirable and water only should be offered as a supplement to milk (even water is unnecessary in exclusively breast-fed babies)
- Healthy foods should be introduced to avoid high-calorie intake and to prime a baby to prefer desirable foods

What young children eat

Anyone working with young children nowadays is aware that they are exposed to many foods that are not good for their health. Research from both the United States and the UK tells us that unsuitable foods are introduced early, and that table foods given to many young children are commonly fast foods that are high in salt and fat, and are accompanied by high-fat and high-sugar snacks and drinks.

Surveys demonstrate that by the time children are 2 years old, 25–30% of them do not eat fruit regularly and the only 'vegetable' they are consuming is chips. Interestingly, a

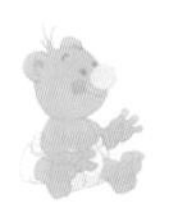

child's intake of fruit and vegetables can be predicted by how long they are breast-fed as a baby, their early eating experiences and their mother's enjoyment of these foods. This gives us some signposts for intervention. The link with later food preferences also occurs in toddlerhood, as studies show that foods preferred between the ages of 2 and 4 years predict a child's food preferences at 8 years of age.

The argument that we need to intervene in the preschool years is strengthened further by research showing that children who eat a junk food type diet at the age of 3 years are more likely to be obese by the time they are 7 years old.

So the way children eat in the preschool years has a significant impact on their diet later in childhood and beyond. It also has a direct link to the development of obesity. If we can develop strategies to improve young children's diets, we could affect their propensity to excessive weight gain and all the health risks that follow.

Key ideas

- Many young children's diets are poor in quality, with inadequate amounts of fruit and vegetables
- Improving young children's diets will influence their later food preferences and their risk of developing obesity

How young children eat

As important as *what* children eat is *how* they eat. This is influenced by a number of factors that include:

- family eating patterns, and whether meals are shared or eaten alone
- parents' control over their children's eating and how much they apply pressure, restriction and monitoring of what is eaten
- 'emotional' feeding. when excessive food is offered to calm or comfort a child
- 'instrumental' feeding, when adults provide food (and usually high-calorie food!) as a reward for good behaviour

Until recently most families often ate together. Now it is commonplace for each person in the family to eat whenever they feel like it, and there is often no time set aside for a family to eat together sociably. In many families food is eaten in front of the television, with little opportunity for family interaction. Older children commonly fend for themselves, and are expected to warm up frozen meals in a microwave rather than eat freshly cooked food. These processed foods are often high in fat, salt and calories, and so contribute to an excessive caloric intake. In countries such as France, where the family meal is still an institution, levels of obesity are lower than elsewhere, so it is possible that the lack of emphasis on social eating contributes to the high levels of obesity in the UK.

A significant key to a balanced lifestyle lies in learning to know when one has had enough to eat. Appetite is a delicate balance, and sadly we are masters at overriding the finely tuned mechanisms that ensure a young child eats appropriate amounts of food. Studies have shown that babies left to their own devices regulate their food intake well. If they are given a calorie load between meals they will reduce the amount they eat at the next feed. Over time, however, they learn to eat for social reasons rather than hunger, and our challenge is to learn how to preserve babies' natural responses when they have had enough. Gone are the days when we should be encouraging children to finish up what is on their plates, or telling them that they are lucky to have food when children in other parts of the world are going hungry.

Interestingly, the way mothers feed their children can have an effect on a child's ability to regulate how much they should eat. Some mothers are controlling and even intrusive, while others are more laissez faire, and yet others put effort into restricting what their child eats. Studies have shown that the children whose mothers exercise tight control over what they eat are more likely to be obese, and it is postulated that their natural appetite control has been overridden. They are also more likely to eat when they are not hungry. Perhaps less surprisingly, children of parents who adopt an indulgent feeding style also have a tendency to become obese.

Children are also more likely to eat when they are not hungry if their parents have restricted them from eating certain foods – such as withholding dessert if the vegetables have not been eaten. The desire to eat these withheld foods is increased, and the opposite effect is achieved than that intended by their parents.

Many people eat for reasons other than hunger. To some extent almost all of us eat for comfort, though this is more true of some individuals than others. It is interesting to reflect on whether this emotional eating is programmed by our parents' use of food for comfort. Babies are commonly offered food as the first response to crying, without attempts to settle the baby through other means. This continues into childhood when sweets are proffered for pain – whether for a cut knee or for feeling miserable. Might we reduce comfort eating later in life by helping parents to find other forms of comfort for distress?

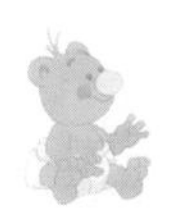

The other way that we perhaps present food inappropriately is by using it as a gift or a reward. How often do we reward good behaviour with food? In fact it can be hard to think of anything else. Some schools still give out chocolate or sweets for prizes, too. Yet there are numerous other ways to reward children.

One of our challenges is to try to influence a long-term change in eating behaviour, and we need to consider how we might achieve this. Could we reintroduce mealtimes where families eat away from the television? Can we encourage parents to respect children's own cues that they have eaten enough, and can we find alternatives to food for alleviating distress and as rewards?

Key ideas

- Family mealtimes are a valuable institution that can help avoid excessive intake of food
- If we learn to respect infants' cues that they have had enough to eat, they will develop the ability as children to respect their own feelings of fullness
- We need to develop alternatives other than food to comfort children – and ourselves
- We need to find treats other than food to reward children – and ourselves

Children's activity levels and television

Obesity results not only from a nutritional intake in excess of needs, but also from a decrease in energy output. Children are clearly less active than they have been in the past, and sadly, studies have shown that nursery age children are also very sedentary, with a direct impact on their risk for obesity. Three-year-olds who watch more than 8 hours television a week are more likely to be obese by the time they are 7 years old than those who watch less. (Those who sleep less than 10½ hours at night are also more likely to be obese – maybe because they are fed at night to stop them crying.)

Many children have independent access to television, and so have little supervision over what they watch. A study in the United States showed that as many as 75% of children beyond the age of 8 have a television in their bedroom, and 36% of very young children do too. Although we do not have exact figures for the UK, the prevalence of television in children's bedrooms is also high.

Surveys of older children show a real dependence on the screen – an average of 2 to 5 hours each day. Some 44% of school-age children use computers every day, and 36% play video games. In fact children spend more time watching TV or playing on a computer than they do in any other single activity except sleep.

Why does television have such a powerful influence on children's development of obesity? Four explanations have been given:

- It replaces physical activity with very sedentary behaviour
- Metabolic rates decrease when watching TV: viewing is associated with lower metabolic rates than any other activity – almost as low as sleeping
- There is a tendency to snack, almost unconsciously, when watching TV
- Junk-type foods are often bought in response to advertisements, and young children's pester power is harnessed by the food industry

Key ideas

- Children of all ages watch a great deal of TV and play computer games for hours at a time
- The more TV that is watched, the greater the risk of obesity
- Young children who have access to TV in their bedrooms are more likely to be obese
- Watching TV increases children's risk of obesity by reducing their physical activity and metabolic rate, and indirectly by increasing caloric intake

What increases children's risks of obesity?

There are a number of factors that increase a baby's risk of obesity. The most important are familial, though socioeconomic factors also play a part, as do a baby's weight and their pattern of weight gain. Despite popular belief, identifiable genetic, metabolic or hormonal causes are very rare.

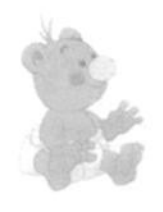

Obesity runs in families, and the debate continues about the extent to which it is caused by genetics or the shared home environment. There is no doubt, however, that the strongest risk factor for obesity is the parents' obesity, and beyond that a wider family history. Figures suggest that if one parent is obese the child has a 40% chance of becoming obese themselves, and if both parents are obese this increases to 80%. Many parents acknowledge this, and are particularly motivated to ensure that that their children do not suffer as they have done.

Another worrying factor is maternal obesity during pregnancy. Research suggests that the mother's weight during pregnancy influences the baby's later weight gain. This provides a clear message that family planning should ideally involve the mother reaching a healthy weight before she becomes pregnant.

However, parents give their children not only the genes that contribute to body size and shape, but the home environment too. If parents are obese, children are at higher risk because of both of these. As we cannot do anything about babies' genetic heritage, the focus of our work must be on helping parents adjust the home environment for themselves and for their children.

Ethnicity also has a part to play. Some ethnic groups are particularly prone to develop obesity, and the health problems (or morbidity) that result. The Hispanic population in the United States and the Asian and black communities in the UK are examples where this is the case. In general it seems that the problem occurs when they adopt a Western diet and lifestyle. Their bodies appear to be even less able to cope with these excesses than those of us who have lived in the West for generations.

Poverty is the other major factor that has an influence on obesity in a community. Disadvantaged children are at higher risk than their more affluent neighbours. It is undoubtedly harder to have a healthy lifestyle in circumstances where fruit and vegetables are expensive and less available, where there are fewer playspaces and where it is more dangerous to be outside without adult supervision.

What helps to reduce obesity

An inadequate amount of research has been carried out on how to prevent or treat childhood obesity. Most of it has focused on strategies to prevent obesity at school, and there is much less evidence on how to help children who are already obese. There is no evidence for very young children and babies, and even that for older children is very limited. Studies have involved only small numbers of mainly primary school aged children, and have on the whole been carried out in specialist centres with highly qualified and experienced staff. The families have been mostly white, middle class and motivated, so it is hard to apply the methods and results more broadly to families living in the UK, particularly those from disadvantaged backgrounds.

Although the programmes themselves may not be directly relevant to all practitioners, the research highlights some important principles that can guide us in working with obesity, which are listed in the table below. It is clear that it is less effective to focus on diet or physical activity alone, and a holistic approach that combines activity with nutritional advice and social support is more likely to be helpful. Second, parents must be involved in the process. Although this may be self-evident for younger children, it is also important for teenagers. Lastly, there is no quick solution – any intervention must be of adequate duration and involve frequent contact and support.

PRINCIPLES FOR EFFECTIVE WORK IN OBESITY

Evidence-based principles	Skills and qualities
Multifaceted approach	Respect
Change in lifestyle	Warmth
Increase in physical activity	Empathy
Decreased sedentary activity	Genuineness
Behavioural contracting	Attentive listening
Nutritional advice	Empathic responding
Social support	Knowledge of healthy lifestyles
Parental involvement	Understanding obesity
Frequent appointments	
Adequate duration	

An additional line of research provides us with further information that is helpful in guiding our input. This comes from studies on parents' opinions about the sort of help they have received for an obese child. We learn from them that although some GPs, health visitors and practice nurses are sympathetic and supportive, parents too often feel blamed and guilty. They also encounter attitudes that make them feel they are making an unnecessary fuss, and are commonly and inappropriately told that their child will grow out of their excess weight. When advice is given it is often dogmatic or dismissive, and does not take family circumstances into account.

Endword

Recent research findings provide a clear message that the early years are a crucial period, as this is when lifestyle habits are developed. Infant feeding, family lifestyle and most

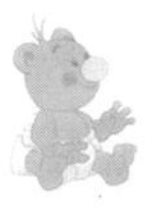

importantly parenting style can influence children's weight and health in the very long term. There is clearly a need for a focus on the first years of life when trying to prevent or reverse obesity.

Happily, research also provides some direction as to how we might work more effectively to help children acquire a healthier start to life. The messages are clear, and a combination of skills and knowledge is needed to deliver these effectively. Above all, practitioners need to be able to engage with parents and carers through respect, warmth, empathy and genuineness, as well as attentive listening and responding.

HENRY has been developed using these principles to tackle obesity by helping parents address the key lifestyle areas – parenting, eating patterns, nutrition, activity and emotional wellbeing. In the following chapter we describe the HENRY approach, including the Family Partnership Model that underpins it and the strengths-based and solution-focused support it offers.

References, further reading and resources

Baird J, Fisher D et al Being big or growing fast: systematic review. *BMJ* 2005; 331: 929

Birch L and Dietz Wi (eds) *Eating behaviours of the Young Child – prenatal and postnatal influences on healthy eating* American Academy of Pediatrics 2008

Bluford DA, Sherry B et al. Interventions to prevent or treat obesity in preschool children: a review of evaluated programs *Obesity* 2007 15: 1341–2

Campbell KJ, Hesketh KD. Strategies which aim to positively impact on weight, physical activity, diet and sedentary behaviours un children from zero to five years: a systematic review of the literature. *Obesity Reviews* 2007. 8:327–338

Edmunds LD, Mulley B et al. How should we tackle obesity in the really young? *Archives of Disease in Childhood* 2007; 92 (suppl 1) A75

Mennella JJ, Jagnow CP et al. Prenatal and postnatal flavor learning by human infants. *Pediatrics* 2001; 107:E88

National Institute for Health and Clinical Excellence *Clinical Guideline* 43 Obesity Guidance 2006

Owen CG, Martin RM et al. Effect of infant feeding on the risk of obesity across the life course: a quantitative review of published evidence *Pediatrics* 2005 115: 1367–1377

ReillyJJ, Armstrong J et al. Early life risk factors for obesity in childhood: cohort study. *BMJ* 2005. 330: 1357–1359

Reilly JJ, Methven E et al. Health consequences of obesity *Archives of Disease of Childhood* 2003. 88: 748–752

Rhee KE, Lumeng JC, Appugliese et al Parenting styles and overweight status in first grade. *Pediatrics* 2006; 117:2047–2054

Robinson TN. Television viewing and childhood obesity. *Pediatric Clinics of North America 2001, 48,* 1017–1025

Rudolf MCJ. The obese child. *Archives of Disease in Childhood Educ Pract Ed* 2004; 89:ep57–62

Speiser P, Rudolf MCJ et al. Consensus development: childhood obesity. Journal of Clinical Endocrinology and Metabolism 2005. 90(3): 1871–1887

Summerbell CD, Ashton V *et al.* Interventions for treating obesity in *The Cochrane Library*, Issue 1. John Wiley and Sons Ltd 2004

Websites

World Health Organisation Growth References
www.who.int/childgrowth/en

Obesity Care Pathway/Your Weight, Your Health Department of Health 2006 www.dh.gov.uk/Publications

The Child Health Promotion Programme Department of Health 2008
www.dh.gov.uk/Publications

Healthy weight, healthy lives – a cross strategy for England Department of Health 2008
www.dh.gov.uk/Publications

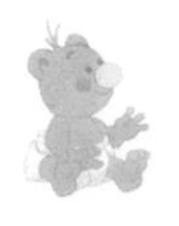

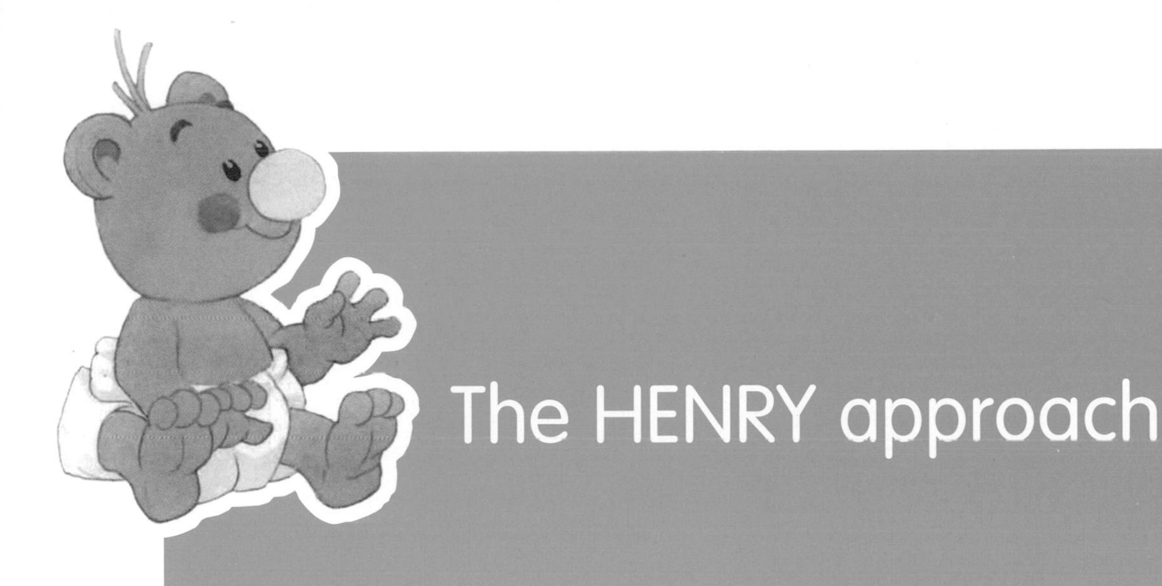

The HENRY approach

2

A baby or young child grows up surrounded by adults – parents and carers, their friends, extended family, staff in childcare settings, and other community practitioners such as health visitors whose role is to support the family. The HENRY approach to preventing and tackling child obesity is relevant to us all. As mentioned in Chapter 1, the principles for effective work in child obesity include a holistic view that recognises the importance of emotional wellbeing and the broader aspects of parenting and parent support, as well as the more traditional topics of nutrition and activity. All these have been incorporated into the HENRY approach.

The approach has three essential elements, which are introduced in this chapter and applied to healthy lifestyle issues in Chapter 3. These are:

- the Family Partnership Model
- solution-focused support
- the need for reflective practice

The Family Partnership Model

The HENRY approach is underpinned by the Family Partnership Model, a highly regarded and well established model for parent support. The name reflects its two core principles: first, that the nature of the relationship between a parent and anyone hoping to give them support is in itself important in the helping process; and second, that the most effective kind of relationship for this work is a partnership. The model offers a way of working with families whatever their reason for needing support, including the question of child obesity prevention and healthy lifestyle promotion.

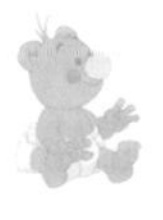

The model is shown below, with each box denoting an important element in the helping process.

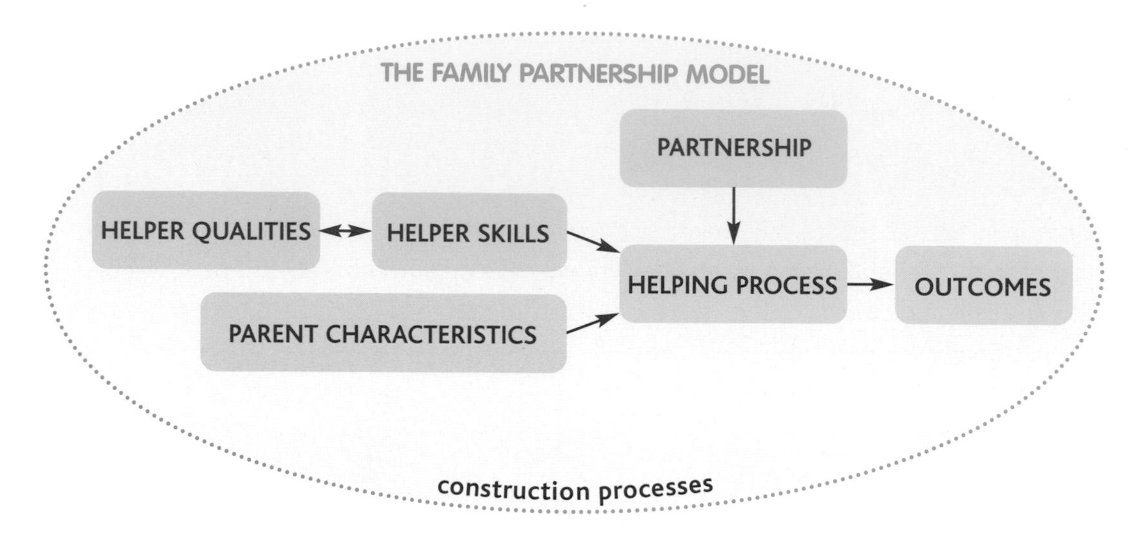

The diagram suggests that positive outcomes result from an interactive process that is most effective when the relationship between the parent and the helper develops as a partnership, and that the qualities and skills of both the parent and the helper play a crucial part in the process. The ellipse indicates that these elements are given coherence by a set of general ideas about how people function psychologically.

Construction processes

All of us try to make sense of our world by building a personal model about our experiences. We begin to do this at birth, and continue the process throughout our lives. The model we construct is not an accurate reflection of reality but a unique interpretation of it – and as each person's experience is unique, each person's model will be different.

One reason why making changes in our lives can be difficult is because doing so involves identifying and reviewing some of our underlying assumptions about ourselves and others.

Reminding ourselves that both we and the parents we hope to help will have developed our personal constructs for our own good reasons can enable us to be truly respectful as we explore their issues and together try to resolve them. Part of our role as helpers is to encourage parents to regard themselves as active, independent and effective – to consider themselves in a positive light. These attitudes may initially be significantly different from the personal constructs they have created as a result of past experiences.

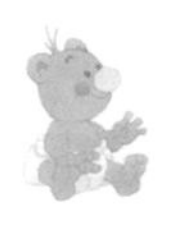

2

Within this framework, the development of a partnership can be seen as two people coming to share constructs about each other and about how they will work together.

Partnership

Relationship building is the most important task within the helping process, so it is important to be clear about the nature of this relationship. The approach identifies the kind of relationship most likely to be effective in bringing about change. There is no guarantee that a helpful kind of relationship will develop automatically. Some types of relationship – such as the expert model, in which the professional is assumed to be the only person with relevant expertise – may be less effective.

There are many possible types of relationship (e.g. friendship, advocacy). In the Family Partnership Model we assume that a partnership is the best approach. However, although the notion of partnership is often used its meaning is seldom defined. We consider the essential ingredients of a partnership to be:

- working closely together with active participation and involvement
- sharing power, with parents leading
- complementary expertise
- agreeing aims and process
- negotiation
- mutual trust and respect
- openness and honesty
- clear communication

Many practitioners are more accustomed to the expert model than to working in partnership. Anyone whose professional training equips them to identify clients' difficulties and problems, rather than looking for their abilities and strengths, can unwittingly reinforce a client's negative attitudes or sense of inadequacy in those they are trying to help. Dispensing advice based on a professional's assessment of a client's needs, rather than the client's own perceptions, can also undermine rather than empower. Truly working in partnership requires us to let the client lead, to follow their agenda rather than imposing our own, and to be a catalyst for change rather than seeking to impose change, however well-meaning our attempts at persuasion!

Participation

An effective helping relationship requires the active involvement of both the parent and the helper. They work together, rather than the helper working on or for the parent.

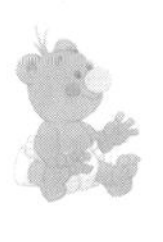

Sharing power
The notion of power is complex in any relationship. Within the model, we assume that partnership involves a notion of equality at least in relation to decision-making. It is most effective for the helper and the parent to share power in deciding what they are doing together, working towards enabling the parent to become the senior partner as soon as possible.

Expertise
A partnership is distinguished from the expert model not by denying the knowledge and skills of the helper, but by fully recognising the expertise of the parent. There is nothing a professional can do, no matter how sophisticated, without engaging the expertise of the parent. Of course helpers also require expertise, and must be able to give appropriate advice and/or treatment. Our notion of partnership requires the expertise of both participants, as positive outcomes are more likely if their expertise is different, complementary and combined.

Agreement
Participants need to come to an agreement about what they are doing together, including their aims and objectives and the ways in which to achieve them.

Negotiation
It is unrealistic to expect people to agree on every issue without discussion, so the notion of partnership is founded on respectful negotiation.

Trust and respect
For a real partnership to develop, the relationship must be based on mutual trust and respect, as people are most likely to work together in this way if they feel respected and safe.

Open communication
Partnership involves sensitive and open communication, so that clear and honest discussion of all the relevant issues can take place.

If partnership is defined by these criteria, it cannot be assumed to develop quickly or naturally, and in some cases may not be achieved at all. A successful partnership will always require time, effort and skill. It will also depend on what the participants bring to the situation, including their commitment and the ability to work in this way.

Developing a partnership will help both to facilitate the subsequent stages of the helping process and to enable positive outcomes. The more the relationship equates to a partnership, and the more involved and open participants can be in exploring parents'

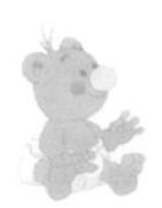

strengths and difficulties, the more likely they are to achieve a useful understanding of their situation, and for problems to be resolved or managed effectively. The more honest participants can be, the easier it is for difficult issues and hidden concerns to be explored. The more control parents are accorded within the relationship, the more their self-efficacy, confidence and independence may be enhanced.

Parents' ability to cope is likely to be increased if they understand the helping process, so the helper needs to be explicit about it. Perhaps the most powerful argument for the development of a partnership is that it may provide a more positive model for parents than they have yet experienced. Not only is their self-esteem likely to improve by their being held in esteem by the professional, but the partnership may also change how they relate to others.

Outcomes

It is easier to help effectively if we are explicit about what we are hoping to achieve. In the Family Partnership Model there are eight general outcomes, whatever parents' issues are and the aims and goals negotiated with them. These outcomes may not always be achievable, but it is useful to keep them in mind.

The outcomes of helping are:

- to do no harm
- to help parents identify, clarify and manage problems
- to enable and empower parents
- to enable parents to foster the development and well-being of their children
- to facilitate the family's social support and community development generally
- to help families access all services relevant to their needs
- to find ways to compensate for difficulties parents or children cannot manage for themselves
- to strive to improve the help we offer and the service systems within which we work

The helping process

The process needed to achieve these outcomes can be thought of as a set of seven interrelated tasks, each building on the one before, as the diagram below shows.

These tasks do not take place in sequence once and for all. For example, while relationship building must always take place first it also continues to develop at every stage throughout the process. The arrow directly from Understanding to Review highlights the

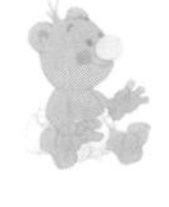

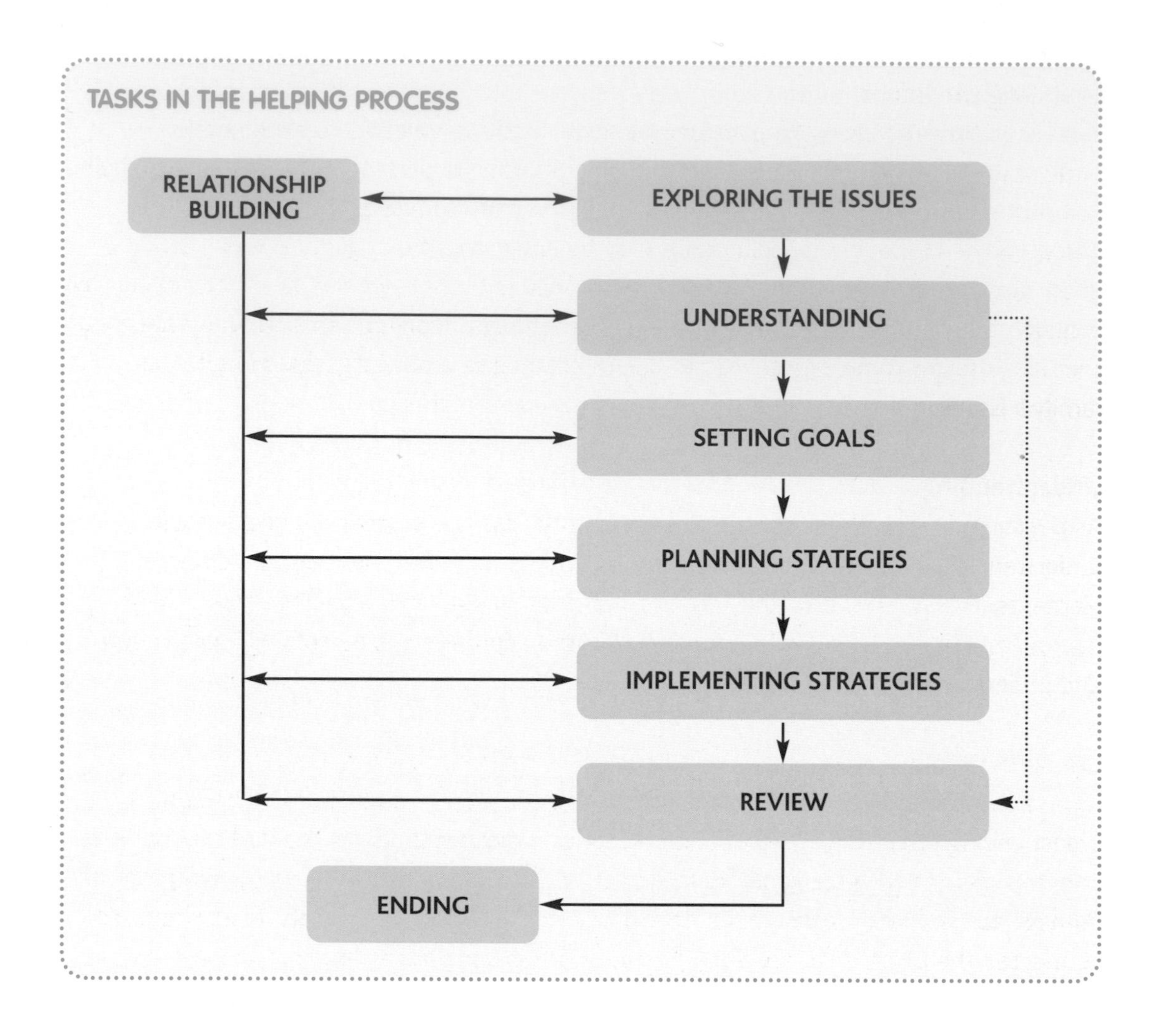

possibility that a better understanding of the problem may be all that parents need – the problem management tasks may not always be necessary. We might also move between tasks at any time: goals, for example, might be adjusted as strategies are planned, and the review of outcomes may result in a return to any of the earlier stages.

Relationship building

The helper's first task is to establish and maintain a good relationship with the parents. This is a complex process that may begin even before they meet (e.g. through correspondence and phone calls). It includes the helper and parent getting to know each other, establishing a degree of trust, and coming to an agreement about what working together will involve. This stage is of the utmost importance, as the quality of the relationship will determine the extent to which the subsequent tasks are undertaken and the overall outcomes are achieved.

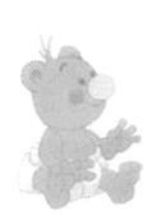

2

Exploring the issues

The second task involves the parents and helper working together to explore the difficulties they have each identified. This begins with the parents' own perspective, their current understanding of the issue, rather than that of the helper. Depending on the nature of the problem, the exploration may be either specific or general. What is important is that it takes place within the parents' own framework. The exploration always includes the important role the helper has in enabling the parents to think carefully about their situation; it is not limited to the helper's formal or informal assessment of the family's issues.

Understanding

As a result of the exploration, the aim of this third task is to achieve a clear, usable understanding of the family's difficulties. This might include identifying the different elements involved and how they relate to each other, and trying to understand their underlying causes. If the exploration is facilitated appropriately, parents will gain clarity and understanding without the need for the helper to offer direct explanations.

During the exploratory stages, it often becomes apparent that a presenting problem is more a symptom than a cause of a parent's difficulty. For example, while exploring a breastfeeding problem with her health visitor one mother suddenly realised that her real concern was not with the problem itself, but with the thought that it was a symptom of damage to the child resulting from the birth. Another mother burst into tears when she connected the onset of behavioural problems in her son with a deterioration in the relationship between herself and her husband. A third came to realise that she had been responding to most signs of distress in her child by feeding him, rather than finding other ways to comfort him. It is by listening to the parent, helping them to tell their story, that these underlying links can be made.

Setting goals

Once there is a clear understanding of the difficulties, parents and helper can move on to the next task: finding solutions. This first needs a joint exploration of what the parents are hoping to achieve so that general aims can be identified. It is often useful to agree explicit goals that are as specific as possible, and that are measurable, realistic and achievable within reasonable time limits. This requires discussion; we should not assume that there will be agreement either among family members or between the parents and the helper about what they hope to achieve.

Planning strategies

The next task is to help parents find suitable strategies to meet their goals. It is essential to involve the parents in the process rather than strategies at once being proposed by the helper with the parent being expected to comply. There are three reasons for this: parents

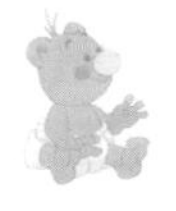

are likely to think of potentially effective solutions themselves; their confidence and self-efficacy will increase; and the experience will help them learn more about the process of finding solutions to issues in their lives. The task here is to think up as many options as possible and then together to choose those most likely to be effective. It increases the chances of success if the selected options are carefully planned with the parents. The idea here is to foresee possible obstacles to the plans and to avoid them if possible.

Implementing strategies

Once strategies have been carefully planned, parents can be encouraged to put them into practice. If parents are well prepared and motivated, and potential barriers have been anticipated, then implementation may be straightforward. Nevertheless, it may help if they feel supported by the helper and able to make contact if necessary.

Review

After an agreed interval, the outcomes of putting strategies into practice are reviewed and their success in meeting the goals evaluated. If changes are taking place, these can be reinforced through recognition and encouragement; if there are difficulties, exploring what happened and why may lead to a deeper understanding, to setting new goals and/or identifying new strategies to try – in other words, a return to earlier stages in the helping process. In either case, there will be the opportunity to learn both from successes and any problems that may have arisen. Sooner or later the time will come to decide that the next step is to end the helping process if all relevant issues have been resolved, making sure that the parents' role in the process is fully acknowledged and appreciated.

Ending

This final task in the helping process needs to be as carefully considered as the others. It is not always possible to do this as the parent may choose at any stage to end the helping relationship – for example by not keeping an appointment. Ideally, the ending will be discussed beforehand and agreed jointly as an extension of the reviewing process. Endings are often not easy; within the model, they can nevertheless provide useful feedback for both parent and helper.

Helper qualities

The Family Partnership Model identifies seven important qualities in helpers. These are similar to the core conditions for person-centred counselling highlighted by the American psychotherapist Carl Rogers. They differ from skills in that they are internal to the person, and cannot be seen by others unless the helper chooses to show them. It is not the existence of these qualities that enables the helping process, but the client recognising them. If as helpers we have these qualities and are able to demonstrate them in all we do, then trust will develop, with the helper being seen as attractive and believable, as strong

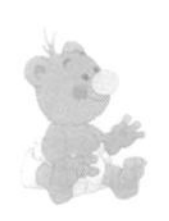

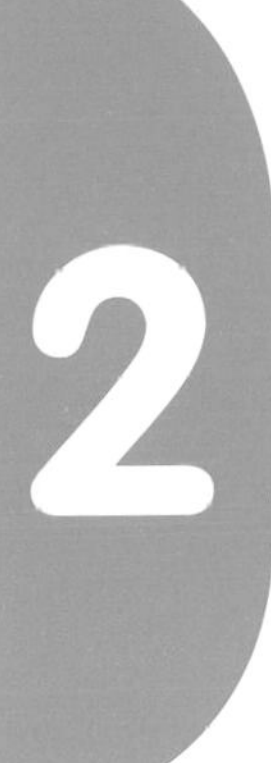

enough to walk beside parents, to validate them, not take over from them, and if necessary sensitively to help them question the paths they might choose to take.

There may be many qualities involved in being effective as a helper. We regard the following as essential:

- respect
- empathy
- genuineness
- humility
- quiet enthusiasm
- personal integrity
- technical knowledge

Each of these represents a set of attitudes or beliefs about oneself and the world.

Respect

This is the first of three characteristics that Rogers regarded as fundamental to therapeutic change. His notion of respect has been understood as meaning warmth, being interested in the client, caring deeply for her/him – having what he called unconditional positive regard. We are in complete agreement with these ideas, and have added one more: a profound belief in a person's ability to cope with their situation, and in their capacity to change.

Empathy

To be effective, Rogers proposed that helpers must have the ability to be open to the experience of the client, to see their problems from their viewpoint without distortion, and then to demonstrate this. This may not always be easy, but indicating to parents that we are really trying to understand them and their situation is the basis for a trusting relationship, open communication, the exploration of an issue – and for change.

Genuineness

This is Rogers' third quality: being honest, unpretentious, non-defensive. With genuineness a helper is open to experience and accurate in viewing situations, as opposed to distorting them for reasons related to his/her own difficulties and defences. This has important implications for how the helper works and is perceived by parents, for the demonstration of empathy and the development of trust.

Humility

Linked to genuineness, this specifically concerns helpers' self-awareness: the need to be realistic and accurate, with an acceptance of our own difficulties and strengths. This quality gives space for the parent to have a role in the helping process. If as helpers we

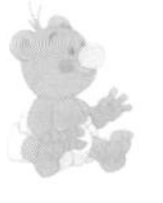

accept that we have limits, and thus avoid both the anxiety that we should have a solution for every problem and the arrogance that indeed we have, we are more likely to seek partnership with parents, actively involving them in understanding situations and finding solutions and constantly eliciting their strengths, resources and expertise.

Quiet enthusiasm

We are likely to be more effective helpers if our efforts to engage with others and listen to potentially distressing circumstances are fuelled by interest, care and even passion. This attitude encourages us to be positive and warm in our interactions with parents without overwhelming them, and provides an impetus for us to continue to improve our skills.

Personal integrity

Related to Rogers' notion of genuineness, this highlights the need for psychological or emotional strength in the helper. We must be able to face the distress of others, be strong for them, and be with them in their difficulties. If we are ourselves distressed or vulnerable we cannot provide the security needed by parents in distress. We need to empathise while remaining able to think independently and differently, and sensitively to offer alternative views to parents.

Technical knowledge

An obvious yet important characteristic is the helper's professional or technical expertise, the array of specialised knowledge and skills acquired through training and experience that supports and extends our innate qualities. Our understanding of the helping processes described in this chapter is included here.

Helper skills

The Family Partnership Model also specifies the skills a helper needs to facilitate the parent–helper relationship effectively. Good communication skills enable us to relate to the parent, to understand the issues they face and to help the parent find solutions that will bring about change.

These skills are:

- attention and active listening
- prompting and exploration
- empathic responding
- summarising
- enabling change
- negotiating
- problem-solving

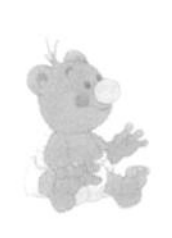

Some of these skills are relevant to every aspect of the process (e.g. attention and active listening); others are limited to particular stages (e.g. problem-solving). It is necessary to understand them – and even more important to be able to use them.

Attention and active listening
This set of skills is the basis of helping and the foundation for the other skills. Effective listening is powerful in engaging parents in the helping process, facilitating partnership, enabling exploration and supporting change. It involves concentrating fully on the parent, filtering all distractions, and watching and listening very carefully in order to hear exactly what the parent says, to notice their tone of voice, facial expression and body language as well as their words, to be aware of what is perhaps not being expressed, and to make sense of the thoughts and feelings evoked by the parent in ourselves. We need to do all this while actively indicating to the person both verbally and non-verbally that we are genuinely trying to understand them.

Prompting and exploration
Listening and attending in themselves prompt people to talk and to explore. There is a range of other skills that can motivate and direct them. These include different ways of responding and prompting, such as open questions ('How did you react to this?') and inviting statements ('I'd be interested to hear more about that'), reflecting back what the person has said ('So you were trying to help him, yet he seemed hurt by what you said'), and allowing time for a reflective silence.

Empathic responding
This is a very powerful way of helping parents to talk, and also indicates that you are truly listening, trying to understand what they are feeling as well as what they are doing and thinking. A simple statement such as 'You sound sad about it' may bring relief to the person simply through feeling understood, enabling them to explore the issue further, and perhaps even to release some intense feelings.

Summarising
Summarising what the parent has been saying is also powerful, and may have similar effects to empathic responding in demonstrating and checking understanding. It may also help to simplify and clarify a complex situation, providing a view that the parents have not considered before, and making it easier for them to explore the situation further.

Enabling change
The process of helping is intimately concerned with enabling parents to change how they perceive and adapt to problematic situations. Change may involve simply being clearer about a situation. It can also include parents thinking differently when they may be stuck or have ideas that are not helpful to them (e.g. being excessively negative about

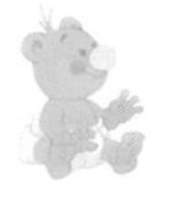

themselves or misinterpreting their children's behaviour). The skills involved in enabling change begin with listening carefully to what people say; summarising their current views in a positive and non-threatening way, asking permission to challenge their views; and then respectfully offering an alternative. This needs to be presented tentatively, as an invitation to the parent as a possibility to consider, not as a certainty or the truth.

Negotiating
Negotiation refers to the process of joint decision-making, or reaching agreement whether or not there is conflict. It is the cornerstone of partnership. As with enabling change, negotiation should reflect a genuine respect for parents, encouraging them to present their views first, and then together comparing and evaluating the different ideas with the aim of reaching a joint decision about them.

Problem-solving
Problem-solving skills overlap considerably with the skills already described. Listening and prompting again provides the basis, with empathy, summarising, enabling change and negotiating decisions about priorities, aims, goals and strategies. At this stage it is also helpful to encourage parents to think creatively about possibilities, to use their imagination, to suspend logic if necessary, and hence to consider as many options as possible.

Solution-focused support

The client-centred approach to therapeutic change was an innovation when Carl Rogers first outlined it in the 1950s. A more recent advance in therapeutic work, which also originated in the United States, is that of solution-focused brief therapy. Solution-focused support is the second crucial element in the HENRY approach.

The principles of solution-focused work sit comfortably alongside the Family Partnership Model, and are similarly relevant to practitioners working to promote a healthy lifestyle in families with young children. They have been included within the HENRY approach because they provide a practical way of helping practitioners resist the temptation to advise parents rather than empowering parents to identify their own solutions. Solution-focused support can have a dramatic effect on parents' belief in their ability to change. When we believe we can do something, actually doing it becomes very much easier.

Solution-focused support

- highlights strengths rather than weaknesses
- identifies what is going well rather than what is not
- is future-oriented rather than examining the past

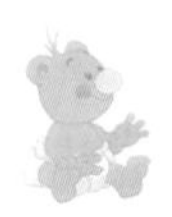

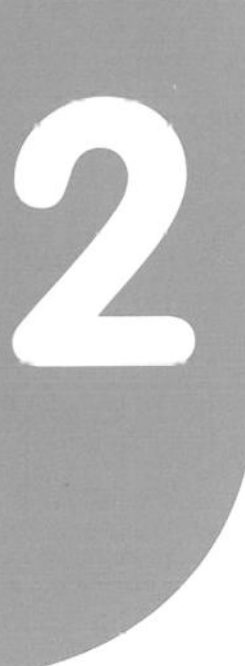

- harnesses parents' knowledge and expertise
- empowers parents to find their own motivation to change
- enables parents to 'rehearse' the changes they will make
- harnesses positive emotions to support behaviour change
- boosts parents' self-esteem and self-efficacy
- releases helpers from the expectation that they need to have all the answers to others' problems

Solution-focused support specifically identifies and highlights the existing strengths and expertise of an individual, focusing on all that they are already doing and using this as a springboard for change. Rather than examining issues and difficulties so that both helper and parent become ever more expert in the details of a problem, the first step in solution-focused support is to focus attention on exceptions to the problem. For example, a parent who seeks help to deal with their toddler's tantrums would be invited to identify times when the toddler is co-operative, and to explore in detail what is happening at these times – places and circumstances when the child is calm, what the parent is doing, what parent and child are feeling when all is going well between them. The second step is to help the parent recognise that they already have the expertise they need, and the third step follows naturally: how to apply these skills more often.

Described thus, solution-focused support sounds simple, and indeed it is – in principle. In practice, it is for most practitioners a fundamentally different way of working. Chapter 3 describes in more detail how to work in a solution-focused way when helping parents adopt a healthy lifestyle for themselves and their families.

Reflective practice

There are two areas in which reflective practice makes a difference to the effectiveness of our work in promoting healthy family lifestyles and tackling child obesity. One of these is personal, the other professional.

To work with integrity in this area, we need to consider our own lifestyle as well as that of the parents we support. One challenge for professionals is that we reflect the population as a whole when it comes to being a healthy weight, overweight or obese, and many of us would benefit from adopting some of the principles and strategies of the HENRY approach. Indeed, many practitioners who attend HENRY training courses do make changes for themselves and their families. Acknowledging the challenges we encounter in doing this helps us both to be more empathic towards parents and more honest in our dealings with them.

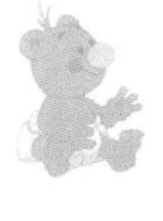

This is not to say that we cannot begin to support parents until we ourselves are an optimally healthy weight, constantly follow healthy eating guidelines, exercise often, regulate our emotions and have succeeded in balanced our work with the rest of our lives! It does mean that we may need to review our own lifestyle and start to make changes that take us in a positive direction. We hope that everyone interested in exploring the HENRY approach will take advantage of this opportunity to reflect on our own lives, and where necessary to put principles into practice for ourselves.

The second way in which we need to be reflective practitioners can both improve the way we work and help us gain a better understanding of the challenges involved in doing things differently. Practitioners who are trained to give advice may at first feel ill at ease and even deskilled when trying to work fully in partnership with parents (letting them take the lead) and in a solution-focused rather than problem-focused way. Those who are experienced in providing empathic support for parents but are unaccustomed to helping them identify goals and strategies for behavioural change may have a similar reaction. Learning any new skill is likely to involve us in a period of uncertainty, and it is important to notice our reactions to this – to the feelings of discomfort that can arise and how we deal with these, to the desire to slip back into old ways and the frustration or dismay when we do, to the need to be patient as we try to let go of old habits and form new ones. This self-awareness is necessary for ourselves and will stand us in good stead when we are supporting parents through the process of change, too.

Endword

In the HENRY approach the messenger is as important as the message. The skills and attitudes that underpin how we work with parents matter just as much as knowledge of what constitutes a healthy lifestyle. In this chapter we have looked at the skills we need; in Chapter 3 we will explore how to apply them in promoting a healthy lifestyle and tackling childhood obesity.

References, further reading and resources

Davis H, Day C & Bidmead C. *Working in Partnership with Parents: the Parent Adviser Model* Harcourt Assessment 2002

George E, Iveson C, Ratner H. *Problem to Solution: Brief Therapy with Individuals and Families* Brief Therapy Press 1999

Jasper M. *Beginning Reflective Practice: foundations in nursing and health care* Nelson Thornes 2003

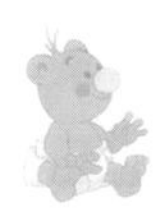

O'Connell B. *Solution-Focused Therapy* Sage 2005

Rogers Carl R. *On Becoming a Person* Constable 1961

Selekman M. *Solution-focused Therapy with Children: harnessing family strengths for systemic change* Guilford Press 1997

Websites

The Family Partnership Model. The Centre for Parent and Child Support
www.cpcs.org.uk

Solution-focused support
www.brieftherapy.org.uk

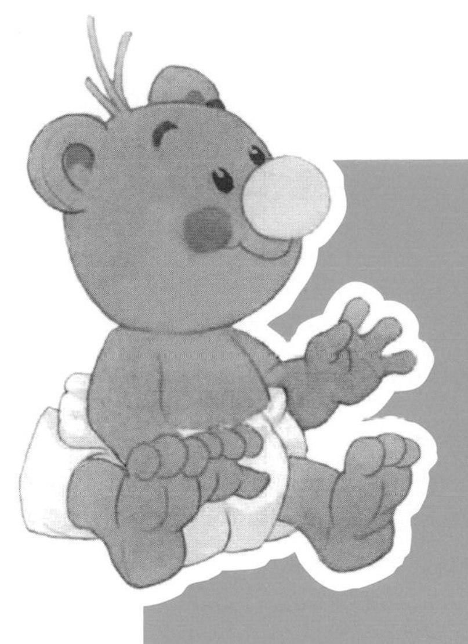

Applying the HENRY approach

3

The purpose of this chapter is to discuss how the HENRY approach can be applied in practice to support families when addressing the problem of child obesity. The principles outlined in Chapter 2 lead to an approach that enables you to:

- explore parents' own understanding of their strengths and difficulties
- undertake an assessment that will help you gain a better understanding of the child, the family and the wider context of their lives
- support parents in setting their goals, and in planning and implementing strategies that will enable them to reduce the risk of obesity and promote a healthy family lifestyle

Because excessive weight gain in infancy and young children has so many factors, simply offering advice on how to manage a child's weight is not likely to be effective. It takes time to understand fully the many issues likely to be contributing to the problem from the parents' as well as from a professional point of view. A principal aim of the approach is to engage parents in the process in a way that supports and empowers them instead of making them feel inadequate in the face of professional expertise. Actively listening to parents' concerns, valuing their strengths, working openly and in partnership with them using a positive, non-judgemental approach, and providing solution-focused support – all these contribute to building self-esteem and motivation, and thus their ability to implement change.

Working in partnership

This approach is somewhat different from the more usual expert or medical model of working, in which the professional is in charge of a consultation, sets the agenda, takes notes, ensures that relevant forms are completed in a logical sequence, etc. There is a shift in control, with the practitioner exercising less and the parent more power over the

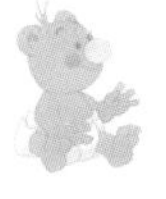

process of exploring their issues and finding ways to resolve them. For many of us, it takes time to become genuinely comfortable with working in partnership, trusting parents to know and understand about themselves and their families, and being more interested in finding this out than in telling them what we think they ought to do. It can be hard to resist jumping in with advice, and to accept that we may be more effective by appearing to do less than we usually do.

In the HENRY approach the professional is used as a sounding board rather than being the person with all the answers, using many skills to manage sometimes difficult situations constructively, empathically and respectfully, encouraging parents' views and ideas, and only tentatively adding suggestions of their own for parents to consider.

The approach outlined in Chapter 2 offers a clear framework for reflection, empowerment and change.

Relationship building

A crucial departure point in the approach is to ensure that time is allowed to establish a positive and trusting relationship. This will sometimes already have happened before the question of unhealthy weight gain comes up; with other families it may be a new contact, and more effort needs to be made to develop the relationship before the sensitive issue of obesity is raised.

Ways of establishing a working relationship will vary with the personality of the individuals. It is likely to involve:

- being genuinely glad to meet the other person/family, and showing this
- being interested in aspects of their life, their home, their child that are not directly related to problems and issues
- offering compliments and appreciation
- finding something in common between yourself and the other person
- sharing something appropriate about yourself
- seeking the other person's ideas and opinions

It can be a real challenge for busy professionals to give time to listen and get to know someone, rather than immediately focusing on problems and offering advice.

When you sense that it is appropriate to move on, it is useful to begin by discovering more about parents' expectations with general questions, such as 'What are you hoping we can achieve?' or 'What are your expectations of me?' This shows interest in their views, and will lay the foundations for working in partnership together. You may be

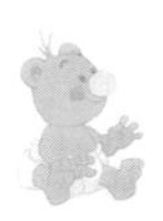

surprised by their expectations of what you can offer, and this is an opportunity to clarify any misconceptions. It also enables you briefly to outline what you think you can offer, and to suggest openly how you think you might work together. Being open about the approach is part of forming an honest relationship with parents; the 'script' given below offers one way of doing this.

INTRODUCING THE APPROACH TO PARENTS

I wonder if it would be helpful to say something about how we might work together. Is that OK with you?

What I'd like to suggest is that we look at what you think the issues are. Once we've done that, we can talk about it to make sure we have the same understanding of what concerns you, and of what you're hoping to gain from me.

The next stage would be to see what you would like to change, and how you might be able to do it. You'll have some ideas, and I might have some ideas for you to think about, too. I'll do all I can to help you put these ideas into practice, and later we will have a chance to see how you have been getting on.

I'm not suggesting that we can do all this at once. How does it sound as a way of looking at things together?

Eliciting information without interrogation involves two key skills: encouraging the other person to talk, and listening well to what they say. Framing enquiries as open rather than closed questions, and including inviting statements rather than only asking questions, makes it easier for the other person to open up (see page 42). When we truly listen to what they are saying, without interrupting, commenting on or challenging what they say, they will tell us even more.

The better we listen, the safer and more respected parents feel. We are also likely to remember more of what they tell us. As it is better to write up notes later, rather than taking them at the time – which may indicate that you are not giving all your attention to the parent – actively listening benefits us as well.

A key element in this approach is to help parents sort out problems in their own minds. By discussing these with a reflective, empathic listener they often gain insights and understanding, work through their emotions, and find new determination to improve the situation.

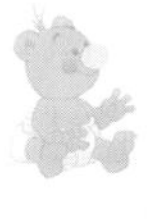

HELPING PARENTS TO TALK

Examples of open questions
When did you first notice this?
What would you like to change?
How often does this happen?
How do you feel about that?

Examples of closed questions
(can be answered just with a 'Yes' or 'No' – often best avoided)
Is this a new problem?
Has he always behaved like that?

Examples of inviting statements
I'm interested to hear more about...
I wonder what ideas you have had about this.
You mentioned...I'd find it helpful if you could say a bit more about it.
Let's see what else you think it might be useful for me to know.

Exploring the issues

The second stage in the helping process involves exploring the parents' concerns. In the context of obesity management, it also covers the need for assessment. All your qualities and skills as a helper will be needed to ensure that the assessment is carried out in a way that both leaves the parent feeling capable (rather than your reverting to the expert model) and tells you what you need to know.

There are many concerns that parents may want to share. They may, for example, be concerned about the effect of the child's weight on their future health and development, or about the type and amounts of food eaten. They may be angry or anxious if there are frequent battles between themselves and a child – over food or in other aspects of family life. There may be a conflict with other adult family members who are undermining what the parent is trying to do. Any of these is likely to be relevant, even if the relevance is not immediately apparent.

Several visits may be needed to gain a full understanding of the issues in the family, and what priority the parent gives to each of these. If practitioners are hasty, with too clear an agenda of their own, they may not discover what really matters to the parent – and are likely to be working at cross-purposes. One of the aims of a first visit is to negotiate with the parents how you see yourselves working together, and to agree a time for a subsequent visit. As highlighted in Chapter 2, it is important to continue to build and

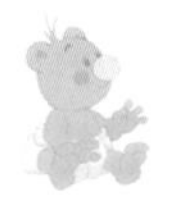

sustain a positive relationship each time you meet; it is not a matter of doing this once and for all!

The main aim of the exploration is to gain a clear understanding both of the parents' strengths and of the difficulties they are experiencing. It is important to focus on parents' strengths – their successes and expertise – and to highlight these in order to avoid giving the impression that for us the parent consists only of a set of problems that need to be solved. The more strengths we can find and appreciatively acknowledge, the more motivated the parent is likely to be, and the more confident they will feel that they can make changes. So time spent on talking about what they enjoy about family life, what they are coping with well, what works in their family, is not time wasted but a valuable investment. These are the attitudes and skills that will support whatever changes are made.

As for the difficulties, some parents will already be concerned about their child's weight gain and actively be seeking help. They are likely to be glad of the opportunity to discuss it, and can be complimented on their concern and readiness to tackle the issue. Others may be dismayed to learn that their child is considered to be at risk. Raising the issue needs to be sensitively handled, as parents are likely to feel criticised or judged. They may blame themselves for the child's weight gain, and question their ability as a parent. Alternatively they may become defensive or even hostile, as your view might challenge a family or cultural norm. If the parents are themselves overweight, sensitivity around the issue may need to be even greater. It is a curious paradox that at a time when obesity levels are rising rapidly, the stigma of being overweight is as great as ever.

Health practitioners tell us that they find it difficult to raise the issue of unhealthy weight in an overweight baby or child, particularly if the parent is overweight themselves. The task may be made easier by using a growth chart to illustrate your concern. Pointing out that the weight is outside the desirable range, or is significantly greater than the infant's length or height, offers an objective observation that can lead on to discussing how this sort of growth pattern can be an indicator of an increased risk for developing obesity. It is even more important for parents to ensure that these children have a healthy start to life. Reassure parents that you are there to help them do this, perhaps emphasising that the messages would be the same for any child – it is just especially important for their baby.

When a parent is already concerned about a child's weight gain, your task is easier. Asking open questions such as 'What are mealtimes like?' or 'Why do you think he/she is putting on weight so quickly?' may encourage parents to talk about their difficulties and help them to think through the problems themselves, and will also allow you to develop a clear picture of what the causes are likely to be. As well as listening well, it is valuable at this stage to check your understanding by offering reflective comments, such as 'It sounds as though you are finding it hard to control what your child eats. Is that right?' Showing empathy allows the parent to see that you are really trying to understand what they are experiencing, so you need to listen at an emotional level too, trying to sense the feelings behind what they describe, and tentatively reflecting these as well with comments such as, 'Mmm, it can be so frustrating when you take the trouble to prepare a healthy meal and the family rejects it. No wonder you are feeling discouraged.'

It is helpful if parents are encouraged to give information in their own way. A formally structured history-taking session suggests that you are more interested in your agenda than in theirs. While it is important to gather all the relevant information, much of this can be achieved by listening, prompting and clarifying where necessary. You may need to ask some direct questions, but only after you have listened well and discovered as much about the family and their concerns as you can by prompting and encouraging the parents to say more, rather than firing questions at them from a pre-prepared list. The list of issues on pages 45 and 46 provides a reminder of the sort of difficulties that may be relevant; it is not intended for use as a box-ticking exercise, which would fly in the face of the HENRY approach.

In some circumstances, particularly if you or the parent are concerned that there are medical or developmental issues, you may need to carry out a more formal assessment. If a partnership has been successfully established, this will not be seen as you focusing on your own agenda. Medical and developmental issues related to obesity are addressed in Chapter 8; it provides details about appropriate assessment, as well as guidance on when referral to other professionals is appropriate.

Understanding

Having established rapport and laid the foundations for a trusting relationship, then listened attentively to the parent and acquired the relevant history, the next task is to summarise the issues that have been aired and to clarify them. Rather than pronounce your own 'diagnosis', it is important to seek parents' views first, then share your thoughts, and finally work out together a summary that makes sense to you both.

There are likely to be several areas to include in the summary, reflecting the complexity of obesity issues. These may include:

- parenting attitudes
- eating patterns
- what is being eaten, and how much
- activity levels
- emotional and behavioural issues
- special circumstances

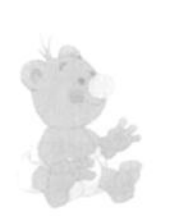

POTENTIALLY RELEVANT ISSUES

The baby/young child

General

- Any concerns about the baby/young child

Eating pattern and appetite

- Early feeding experiences and difficulties
- Patterns of eating – set mealtimes and grazing
- Child's appetite and indication of hunger
- Independence in eating (as appropriate for age)
- Independent access to food
- Use of food for treats, rewards or comfort

Nutrition

- Early feeding: breast or bottle
- Age at weaning
- Foods eaten and usual diet
- Likes and dislikes

Play and activity levels

- Child's preferred activities
- Activity levels
- Amount of TV watched
- Television viewing while eating

Development

- Developmental milestones
- Eating skills – finger feeding, use of spoon, fork, knife and cup
- Motor development – effect on mobility if disordered

Behaviour

- Child's temperament
- Behaviour at mealtimes
- Conflicts between parent and child
- Sleep problems – bedtime or night waking

Medical issues

- Pregnancy/birth/postnatal history
- Medical problems and hospital admissions
- Medication
- Family history of obesity, heart disease and diabetes

The family

- Family members, and who is in the home
- Family eating patterns and enjoyment
- Use of a table for meals, and presence of TV
- Family foods
- Family activities
- Use of food for comfort, treats, bribery and rewards
- Parental attitude to food, any history of eating disorders

Parenting and child care

- General style of parenting: authoritative, authoritarian, indulgent or neglectful
- Child care arrangements and parental satisfaction, especially as regards eating and activity
- Approach to discipline
- Parental mental health (particularly postnatal depression)
- Any parental learning difficulties
- Other influential adults such as grandparents

Social and cultural context of the family

- Accessibility of fresh food close to home
- Religious and other requirements affecting how the family eats
- Opportunities for outside activities and play close to home
- Involvement with an ethnic community
- Financial concerns and employment
- Any involvement with social services, how this was experienced

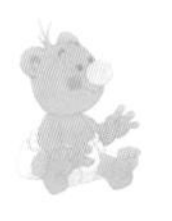

This stage in the process provides a springboard for deciding together what changes are desirable (the goals), and how to go about achieving them (planning strategies and implementation – putting them into practice).

Setting goals

The next task is to work together to identify parents' goals. Change is more likely to take place if parents find their own goals and solutions rather than if these are imposed by the professional. Put your own skills and knowledge at the service of the parent by first encouraging their insights and suggestions, and only then tentatively offering suggestions of your own for them to consider.

The goals need to be explicit rather than general, and need to be achievable. This may involve breaking them down into several small steps rather than one giant leap. If there are several different issues, once these have been identified it is helpful to ask parents what they see as the priority and therefore what they want to tackle first. Some parents, for example, may want to address a specific food issue, while for others general parenting issues are of more concern, and others still may feel motivated to become more involved in playing with a child or introducing more physical activity.

In discussing goals it may become apparent that more information is needed. You may, for example, agree that it would be helpful to observe or record a mealtime, or for the parent complete a food and activity diary for the child that will help you explore dietary and lifestyle patterns in more detail.

Success in one or two easier issues of the parents' own choice will give them the confidence to tackle more difficult problems later on, whereas a parent who is encouraged to attempt too much risks failure and is likely to become disheartened.

Planning strategies

This is the 'how' stage: what is the parent actually going to do differently? What strengths can they draw on to put solutions in place? If the relationship building has been effective, you will have identified parents' strengths and successes, which can be recalled and harnessed to help them initiate change and believe in their ability to see it through.

When there is concern about obesity it is likely that lifestyle change will be a significant element in any actions that are planned. The task may be easier if children are included in the process.

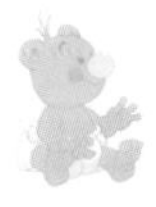

Exploration, understanding, setting goals and planning strategies are all achieved more positively within a framework that highlights existing strengths and helps parents and children to acknowledge these in themselves. Some parents may find it hard at first to identify what they are already achieving, or believe that a professional is interested in this, but gentle persistence using a solution-focused approach will prove a good investment in time and attention. An example of solution-focused support is included at the end of this chapter.

Implementing strategies

This stage is up to the parent. If the earlier stages have been conducted respectfully and in a genuine spirit of partnership, and the goals and strategies are manageable and realistic, you can reasonably hope that the parent will be motivated and confident enough to initiate one or more changes they would like to make.

Part of this discussion may be to agree that you come to observe a mealtime, or when to have a further meeting to see how parents are getting on – the review stage.

Review

When you come to review what changes have been made, and how well they worked, it is worth bearing in mind that breaking old habits and forming new ones is for any of us a considerable challenge. It is important to begin on a positive note, identifying what worked and why and to celebrate changes that have been successful, before going on to explore unresolved issues. Success breeds success, and highlighting what has gone well, encouraging parents to be pleased with what they have achieved, is crucial. What have they learned that will help them to make further changes, or to have another attempt at something that didn't work so well?

It is possible that parents will have done more than was agreed if things have been going well; alternatively, other difficulties (e.g. illness in the family) may mean that there were barriers to changes taking place. It is important to remain supportive and empathic, whatever outcomes the parent reports. This will maintain an atmosphere of trust, and enable the parent to report and reflect honestly on what has happened.

It is likely that the review will also include reflecting on goals and strategies again, and either revising them on the same issues, or moving on to tackle other issues that need to be addressed. It is possible that further exploration may be needed, and greater understanding. In other words, you may need to revisit some or all stages in the process several times before the work is done. Solution-focused support (see below) continues to

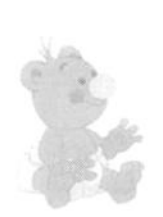

be effective whether the parents' goals have been reached or further work is needed to achieve them.

Ending

The time will eventually come for the intervention to end. Ideally, the timing for this needs to be agreed with the family. If there are multiple difficulties, support may be needed in the long term; with other parents, an initial exploration, some extra information and plenty of encouragement may be all that is needed to set them on the path to a healthier lifestyle for the whole family.

Giving solution-focused support

Working in partnership and giving solution-focused support go hand in hand. The solution-focused approach depends for its effectiveness on three Rs: rapport, reflection and reinforcement.

A solution-focused exchange is given in the example below, which has been included in detail to demonstrate how the process unfolds. Notice the way the practitioner acknowledges the parent's concerns, responds to the parent's ideas and keeps the conversation focused on an easier future.

Solution-focused support

Parent Mealtimes can be such a battle. We all end up in such a state that I dread them sometimes

Practitioner It sounds as though you're having a hard time and are feeling very worried about it.

Parent Yes, I just don't know what to do – I've tried everything.

Practitioner Let's have a think. Imagine there's a scale of 1 to 10, with 1 meaning that mealtimes are a nightmare, and 10 being that they're just fine. Where would you say you are at the moment?

Parent Oh, I should think we're on 2, it's got pretty bad.

Practitioner That sounds really tough. Where would you like to be?

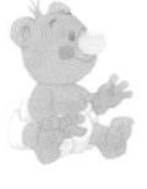

Parent Mmm, about 7 would make a big difference.

Practitioner So being at 7 would be a load off your mind. When you get to 7, how will you feel?

Parent That would be fantastic, though I can't see how to do it.

Practitioner So it'll feel fantastic. What else will you feel?

Parent I think I'd feel proud of myself, and the baby wouldn't be so stressed either.

Practitioner So it will be better for both of you. Let's look at how things are now. What are you already doing to be as high as 2 on the scale?

Parent I hadn't thought like that. Well...I suppose I'm trying to notice food that he likes, and to give him that rather than the stuff he won't eat.

Practitioner So you're spotting what he likes; what else are you doing?

Parent Well, some days are better than others. I think when I'm in a hurry it's harder, so when I'm more organised I don't have to feed him in a rush before collecting the others from school.

Practitioner You seem calmer when you're talking about when it works better! Having more time to feed him really makes a difference – so you've noticed that as well as thinking about what foods to try.

Parent Yes, but it's still difficult because he makes such a fuss and cries and then I get angry.

Practitioner It does sound frustrating. Let's think about how to head towards the 7 you'd like to achieve. What is a realistic next step between 2 and 7?

Parent Maybe 4 would be a good place to get to.

Practitioner That'll be quite an improvement. When you get to 4, what will you be doing differently?

Parent That's quite hard...maybe I could sit and eat something with him, so I'm doing what I need him to do.

Practitioner What a great idea! It can be so helpful if they see us eating too. What else will you be doing?

Parent Well, if I'm eating as well I won't want to hurry him up so much, which might be better.

Practitioner So taking your time will help both of you as well. What do you think you'll notice is different when you're eating with him and going slower?

Parent I think I'll be less impatient and frustrated, and he won't cry so much.

Practitioner That sounds calmer and more comfortable for both of you. What else will you notice?

Parent He'll probably get better at letting me try different foods with him – not just scream whenever I try something different.

Practitioner So you'll be able to try new foods too. And how will you feel about things when this is happening?

Parent It will be easier, and I won't be so worried. It'll be a relief!

Practitioner You look happier about it already. I'll look forward to hearing next time how you're getting on.

The early stages in the helping process will have built up rapport through attentive listening and empathic responses – tuning in to the parent's emotional state. It is in the goal-setting and strategy-planning stages that solution-focused support on any issue really comes into its own. Reflecting on the parent's descriptions of what is already working well, what will be happening when things have improved, and how they will feel about it, all helps to anchor these in the parent's mind, and to turn possibilities into probabilities. Reinforcement through encouragement and praise builds the parent's confidence in their ability to carry out their plans.

Endword

This chapter provides you with a way of putting the HENRY approach into practice when working around changing lifestyle patterns, particularly in relation to obesity. This will involve letting go of an expectation that as the professional you will set the agenda and be in charge. The parent will have more influence over the process of identifying their strengths and choosing the issues they wish to address. You will need to adjust to your

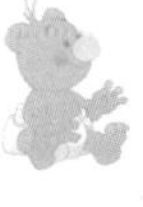

role as a sounding board rather than being the sole repository of expertise and dispenser of advice. With practice the idea of working in partnership with parents and offering solution-focused support will come more easily.

Taking a truly partnership approach is often a challenge for professionals who have been trained in the expert model. It takes skill to manage difficult situations constructively, empathically and respectfully; in this area of behavioural change the approach is likely to be productive and rewarding for parents and practitioners.

References, further reading and resources

Davis H, Day C & Bidmead C. *Working in Partnership with Parents: the Parent Adviser Model* Harcourt Assessment 2002

George E, Iveson C, Ratner H. *Problem to Solution: Brief Therapy with Individuals and Families* Brief Therapy Press 1999

Jasper M. *Beginning Reflective Practice: foundations in nursing and health care* Nelson Thornes 2003

O'Connell B. *Solution-Focused Therapy* Sage 2005

Rogers Carl R. *On Becoming a Person* Constable 1961

Selekman M. *Solution-focused Therapy with Children: harnessing family strengths for systemic change* Guilford Press 1997

Websites

The Family Partnership Model. The Centre for Parent and Child Support
www.cpcs.org.uk

Solution-focused support
www.brieftherapy.org.uk

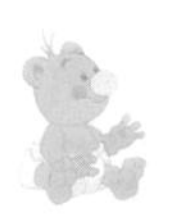

THE HENRY APPROACH IN PRACTICE

PART TWO

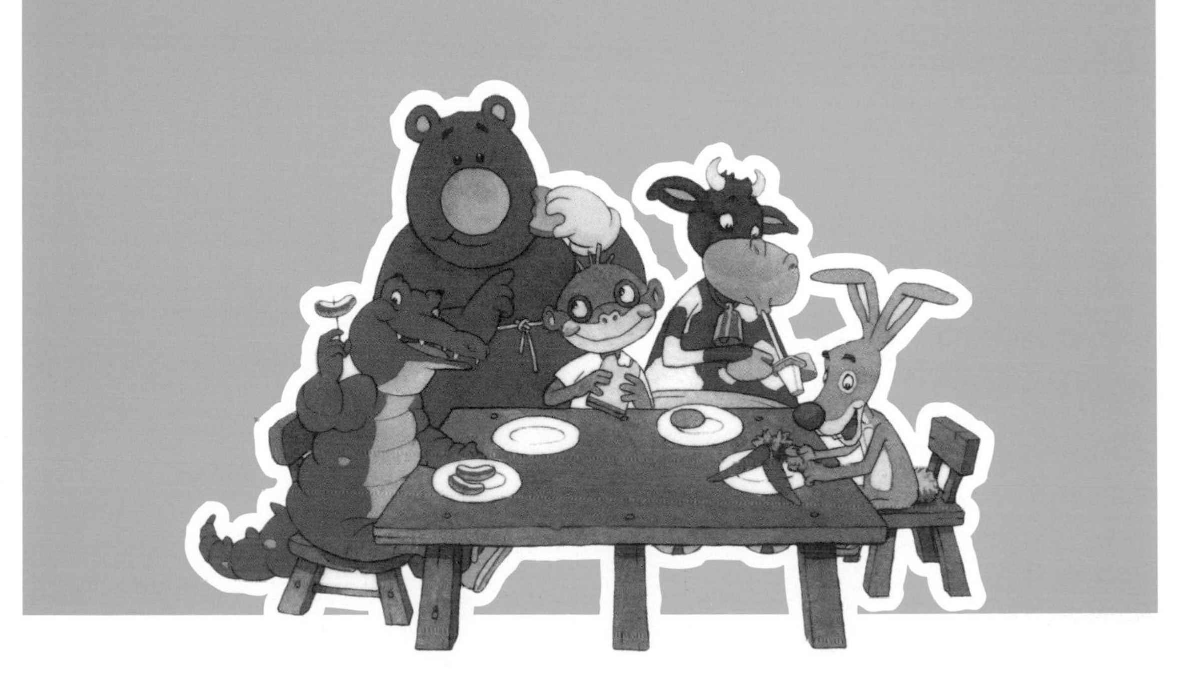

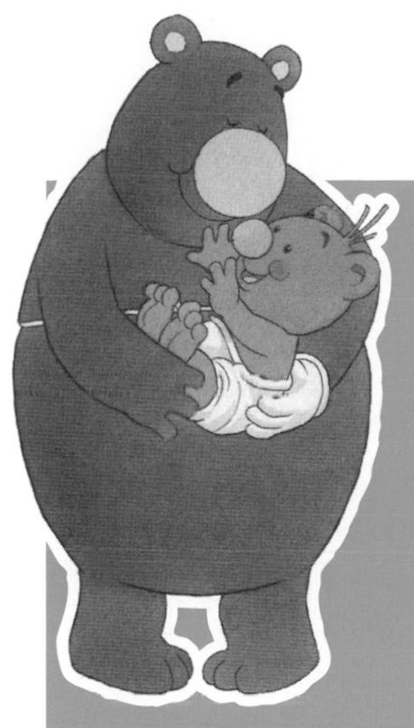

Parenting for a healthy lifestyle

4

Parenting is the key to both preventing and resolving child obesity. Emotional wellbeing, good nutrition and plentiful activity are the pillars which ensure that children are in the best position to cope with any adverse environment. If any of these three elements is excluded or inadequate, the child is exposed to the risk of developing obesity. As children today grow up in a society that promotes an unhealthy lifestyle, helping parents strengthen their parenting skills is more important than ever, and is the most effective strategy we have. This chapter is therefore crucial in preventing obesity in young children, and in the HENRY approach takes first place ahead of healthy eating patterns, nutrition and physical activity.

In this chapter we will explore:

- the role of parenting in establishing a healthy lifestyle
- what influences parents' attitudes
- the baby's need for relationship
- styles of parenting
- positive approaches to parenting
- parents' own needs
- how to promote authoritative parenting

The role of parenting

Parenting is something that many of us spend a large part of our lives doing. It is also something that many parents feel anxious about, perhaps because we recognise that what we do has such a significant influence on our children's development. This is particularly true in the early years of a child's life, when they learn fundamental things about themselves and others, including whether they are lovable and acceptable, whether they can influence the people around them, and whether other people are trustworthy. The

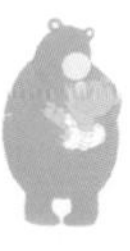

way in which parents convey all this to children is implicit in the way we treat them. Of course, children learn important things about themselves from many people, but in the early years parents are their most important source.

To understand why a baby or toddler is gaining weight too fast, we need to look not only at their eating patterns and the food they eat, but also at the broader parenting that is taking place. Feeding a baby or toddler is, of course, just one of many activities parents undertake to nurture a child and promote his or her development, and a child's attitudes, beliefs and behaviours around food and activity are to a large extent shaped by the parenting they receive.

What influences parenting?

Parenting does not occur in a vacuum. It is influenced by many factors. In the early weeks and months, it is most often the mother who takes on many of the principal tasks of parenting. How comfortably she does this will depend on whether she is mostly happy or mostly sad (her mental health), whether she can provide for her baby (income), whether she feels confident about looking after her baby (self-efficacy) and believes she is a good mother (self-esteem), the amount of support she receives (partner, family, social network), whether she is old enough or mature enough to have addressed her own need to be parented, her awareness of babies' needs, and her views about parenting. These views will have developed according to the way she was parented herself, her cultural and religious background, her social group – and her reflections on all these. These factors are of course also true not only for fathers and other family members but also for the professionals who support parents and care for babies and young children: midwives and health visitors, childminders, staff in nursery settings, etc.

The baby's need for relationship

The distinguished paediatrician D.W. Winnicott once observed that there is 'no such thing as a baby', by which he meant that babies cannot exist on their own. They are from the outset part of a relationship, initially with their primary caregiver (usually the mother), and also part of the broader network of relationships that is their family and community. In addition to basic activities such as feeding and clothing the baby, parents undertake many tasks that are crucial for their baby's healthy development. These include helping them to feel safe, to regulate their emotions, to learn the skills they need, and to find out about the world, their place in it and their relationships with others. These fundamental activities are what we more broadly refer to as parenting, and the way in which parents undertake this role is particularly important.

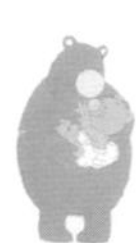

Babies arrive in the world primed for relationship. From birth they show a preference for faces and face-like patterns, and within hours can distinguish and show a preference for their mother's voice, smell and face. Babies quickly develop a sophisticated understanding of facial expressions, distinguishing surprise, fear, sadness, anger and delight, and express this by making corresponding expressions of their own. They look longer at joyful faces than at angry ones, and are sensitive to the emotional nuances in a tone of voice. Before their first birthday they will seek emotional information from others to help them interpret what is going on around them, and their brains will already have developed according to the sort of emotions to which they have been exposed.

The fact that babies are able to make connections between what they do and the response they get primes them to learn from early interactions. The interaction between baby and parent is a key element in this learning. By their first birthday babies have developed internal models of interactions that they have repeatedly experienced during the first year of life. These models are significant, because although they will undergo some reorganisation during the next few years, particularly as the child learns to use language, they will form the basis for the subsequent expectations of himself and others.

4

Healthy self-esteem

Because we form a view of ourselves based on our early experiences in relationship with others, parents who have themselves had unhelpful early relationships may struggle with their self-esteem. That said, many parents who have painful childhood memories are determined to respond differently as parents, and often succeed. Liking ourselves is an important ingredient for liking others, and parents who have a positive attitude towards themselves find it much easier to have a positive attitude to their children. Parents who are highly self-critical may find it more difficult to accept the mistakes and messiness that are an inevitable part of family life.

The key qualities for helpers identified in the Family Partnership Model provide a blueprint for the HENRY approach to parenting as well as to parent support. Parents need to receive high-quality care to help them give high-quality care. If we want to help parents, we need to pay just as much attention to the way we relate to them as we do to how they relate to their children: in other words, we need to practise more than we preach! Having realistic expectations of them, being generous in our praise, building their confidence through power-sharing and choice, and above all being empathic towards them, will help to raise parents' self-esteem as well as modelling helpful ways of responding to their children.

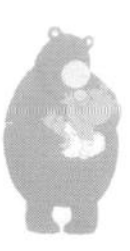

Styles of parenting

Parenting is often taken for granted, but raising a family is in fact one of the most complex and challenging – and long lasting – tasks we ever undertake. Because of this complexity, styles of parenting are not easy to define.

Various models have been proposed to categorise styles of parenting. The one shown below is widely known, and is particularly relevant within the context of promoting a healthy lifestyle as, in addition to identifying different approaches to parenting generally, it has also been linked to feeding styles (see also Chapter 5).

The diagram shows the four major parenting styles, which differ in the extent to which the parenting is more or less responsive to, and more or less in charge of, a dependent young child.

Of course, parents rarely fall precisely into just one category. Most of us vary in our parenting, moving between the different styles depending on circumstances, mood, our own childhood experiences, later role models and influences, and so forth. Parents may adopt a different style in different areas of their child's life – perhaps, for example, having quite an authoritarian attitude at mealtimes while being indulgent when it comes to other aspects of family life such as bedtime. Depending on their personalities, a parent may also have a predominantly different style with different children. Despite these variations, most of us will have general tendencies, and without labelling or judging parents it can be helpful to be aware of these when supporting parents in their parenting role.

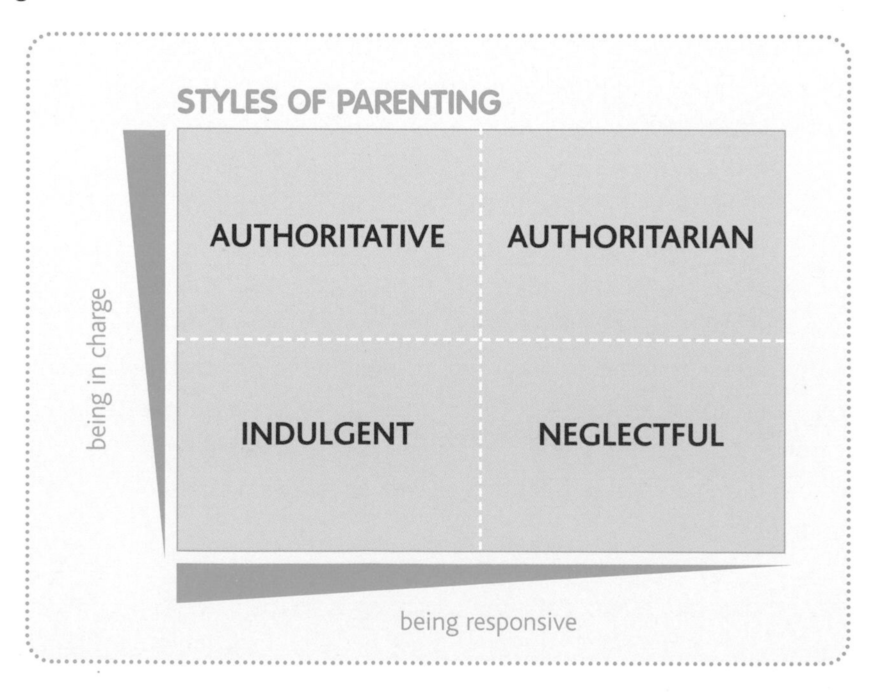

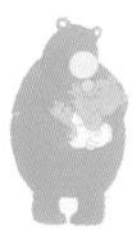

We will look briefly at each of these styles, and then explore in more detail the value of responsiveness within authoritative parenting.

Authoritative style

The ideal style of parenting is one in which the parent is sensitive and responsive to the child's needs, emotions and other cues, and is also clearly in charge with the confidence to establish and maintain appropriate limits or boundaries for behaviour. The authoritative style is the most effective approach to parenting.

It is useful to be clear in our own minds why the authoritative style is most helpful: it promotes the healthy development of the child, who feels secure, knowing that their needs will be respected and their views considered within a consistent framework; a confident and co-operative child is likely to result. This style also makes raising children more rewarding and enjoyable for parents and reduces tension and conflict within the family.

Authoritarian style

When being in charge is taken to extremes, a parent will exercise a high degree of control coupled with low responsiveness, tending towards a parenting style that is very restricting, and demanding compliance from the child without their needs, feelings and preferences being taken into account. A child raised in this way is likely to become anxious and withdrawn or rebellious and defiant.

Indulgent style

This is a kind but weak approach to parenting, in which the parent is responsive to the child's wishes and demands even when these are not in the child's best interests. The parent does not feel confidently in charge, and is unable or unwilling to set limits and maintain boundaries, so every wish is granted and every whim is catered for – the child rules the roost, and may become selfish and demanding.

Neglectful style

A neglectful parenting style differs from the indulgent style in that the parent is neither in charge of nor responsive to the child. The parent may be unaware of the child's needs nor set any boundaries. Carried to extremes, this attitude becomes neglectful. Children may come to believe that their parents do not care about them, and may be confused or resort to extreme behaviour as a way of attracting attention.

The value of responsiveness

One of the most important aspects of early parenting is parents' ability to be sensitive to their baby or young child. As we have already seen, from the very early days of life babies

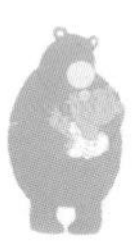

are sensitive to the emotional environment that surrounds them, and learn from the way others respond to them.

Responsive parenting has a number of important components. First, it involves a parent being 'attuned' to the baby or young child both in reading their emotional state and in communicating sensitively. Much of what we know about the way in which parents and babies interact has been obtained by studying video footage of mothers and babies together. What this shows is that the interactions between them take place in a sort of dance. When this dance is interrupted or does not flow smoothly, either the parent or the infant needs to be able to repair it. Some parents are very skilled at this. When the parent and baby have been engaged with one another, the baby may feel the need to look away, disrupting their engagement. A sensitive parent will accept this break, and wait comfortably until the infant is ready to re-engage.

Other parents are either not able to engage their baby in the dance, or are not able to repair it when it is interrupted. Such parents are on the whole either too intrusive for their infants or insufficiently engaging. In the example just given, they may experience the infant's need for a break as rejection, and refuse to accept the disengagement, continuing to try and get the baby's attention. Mothers who are withdrawn, perhaps as a result of postnatal depression, are often unable to engage the infant in the dance, or to maintain it.

Another important component of sensitive parenting is a parent's ability to recognise and relate to her baby as having intentions and desires of his own – being an individual in his own right. Babies of mothers who can do this show better later development.

A baby with parents who are repeatedly able to engage in a mutually satisfying series of exchanges learns to expect mutually rewarding relationships with others. They learn that their feelings and needs will be respected, and are able to engage with the parent (and with others) in a satisfying way. Infants with parents who are intrusive may come to expect this of other relationships, learning that their feelings or needs will not be respected, and that relationships are fraught with problems. The insecurity that results often leads to later behaviour problems, both within the family and beyond (e.g. at nursery and later at school). Infants of parents who are withdrawn or disengaged may also learn that relationships are unsatisfying and that their needs will not be met; they too may become anxious, depressed, withdrawn or angry.

Mirroring

Another aspect of responsive parenting is parents' the ability to 'mirror' the baby's emotional state. This might involve adopting a sad face and murmuring in a gentle way to show their understanding when the baby is feeling sad or unhappy, or smiling warmly when the baby smiles and saying cheerfully how happy they look. This capacity for

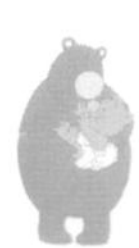

empathy, for tuning in to and reflecting the infant's emotional state, is a valuable skill that supports a close relationship throughout childhood – and beyond. Emotional attunement is the first stage in the child's ability to develop empathy for others – one of the key components of emotional literacy and a cornerstone in establishing close and satisfying relationships throughout our lives.

Empathy is not always easy to provide even when we are in an emotionally neutral state ourselves. When any of us is overwhelmed by our own emotions, in the way that angry, anxious or depressed mothers are, it is particularly difficult to identify or respond appropriately to a baby's feelings.

Containing emotions

Another important component of responsiveness is the parent's ability to help a baby or young child learn to regulate their emotional state by acting as a 'container' for the raw emotions they express. Some parents – perhaps anxious, depressed or angry – may be overwhelmed by the baby's feelings and behaviour, and unable to respond in a way that helps to contain them, or be so overwhelmed by their own emotions that they remain unaware of those the child is experiencing. These babies and young children are not only left with their own raw and unregulated emotions, but need to deal with the adult's unmanageable feelings as well. A calm and sensitive parent might, on the other hand, gently and firmly rock a screaming, frustrated baby, while talking calmly to reassure them. This containment from another is the first step in the baby learning how to regulate their own emotions as they develop and mature.

Parental modelling

A different kind of mirroring takes place as children grow and develop. They themselves become a mirror, reflecting the attitudes, behaviour, gestures, language, beliefs and emotions of those around them. One of the first words in many children's vocabulary is 'No!' This is often given as an example of toddlers' typically rebellious behaviour, but it is worth pausing to ask ourselves whether they learn the word so early because it is one they often hear. A 3-year-old who swears is likely to be reprimanded at nursery, but where do they pick up the vocabulary? A child who is kind, or another who laughs, when someone is hurt, will be copying the most common reaction they have experienced themselves or noticed in others. The examples are endless. A child learns readily to do what we do; it is much harder for them to do as we say!

This copying process is of course also true in relation to the family's lifestyle. If parents are modelling healthy attitudes to food and activity – being sociable at mealtimes, enjoying trying new foods, eating a range of healthy foods with relish, being physically active – the child will without knowing it be absorbing these messages and will be likely to adopt the same attitudes.

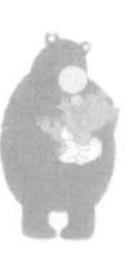

Key ideas

- parenting plays a vital part in establishing a healthy lifestyle and preventing obesity in babies and young children
- parenting attitudes are shaped by personal experiences and wider influences
- babies and young children have a highly developed need for relationship
- healthy self-esteem in the parent is important for responsive parenting
- an authoritative parenting style is the most helpful approach
- empathic attunement, mirroring and containment provide optimal conditions for a baby's emotional development
- babies and young children are imitators: they absorb and copy the attitudes and behaviour of the adults around them, particularly their principal caregivers

A positive approach to parenting

Adopting a positive approach stands parents in good stead at every stage of childhood. There are some key ideas and strategies that can make the demanding, frustrating and wonderful job of being a parent easier. In the HENRY approach we have selected those that also contribute to promoting a healthy family lifestyle.

Parents' needs

A crucial and often neglected aspect of parenting is for the parents' own needs to be met. Some parents feel uncomfortable when they are encouraged to do things for themselves, saying that they do not have the time or money, or that it seems selfish and they feel guilty. But none of us can continually give our attention, energy and time to others without recharging our own batteries. In other words, parents deserve to adopt the same sensitive, responsive approach with themselves as the one that is recommended for parenting. It is when we neglect ourselves, or expect ourselves to keep going for days or weeks on end without a break, that we are likely to lose patience with young children, neglect their needs, collapse in front of the TV rather than engaging in activity, or resort to comfort eating.

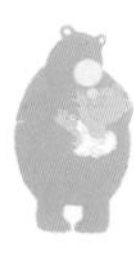

Encouraging parents to take good care of themselves is an effective way of helping them take good care of their children. In addition, in their own right parents deserve to look after their own needs physically, mentally and emotionally. Healthy food and regular physical activity, spending time with other adults, enjoying ourselves and having small treats all contribute to the sense of well-being we need to enjoy family life. Helping parents to recognise this, and perhaps to notice more often what they are already doing for themselves, can make a real difference to their (and our!) zest for life.

SOME WAYS PARENTS CAN MEET THEIR OWN NEEDS

- parent swap – looking after someone else's child for an afternoon, and then having an afternoon free
- spending time enjoyably with partner
- sitting down to drink a cup of tea
- having a peaceful scented bath
- buying a bunch of flowers
- joining a parent and toddler group – company for both parent and child
- listening to music
- buying a magazine – and reading it
- spending time with friends
- doing sport or other activities

Realistic expectations

Some parents have little idea of what to expect of a baby or a toddler. Many of the conflicts that arise – over a baby repeatedly dropping a spoon on the floor, or a toddler's fascination with electric sockets, for example – arise because the behaviour is interpreted as 'naughtiness' when it is in fact developmentally normal. Much of a toddler's frustration may be the result of their needing more independence than their parents recognise. Helping parents acquire a clearer idea of their children's developmental stages in the early years will help them be more realistic, and allow them to encourage a young child's gradual need for autonomy in a safe and supportive environment,

Empathy

We have already described the importance of empathic attunement from the earliest days of a baby's life. This is not easy, and is particularly hard to manage when we are in the grip of our own emotions. Learning to be more self-aware and to be empathic towards ourselves can help us become more sensitive and accepting of others, too.

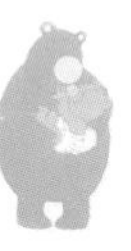

Setting ourselves on one side and really trying to understand a situation from someone else's point of view remains one of the most important skills of responsive parenting – indeed, of any relationship. Empathy is also a valuable first step in managing a young child's behaviour. Understanding and responding to how they are feeling can help a parent avoid many of the situations that lead to difficult behaviour. As parents, it can help us stay gentle with a baby who is screaming with hunger, and calm with a toddler whose numerous minor frustrations have accumulated to the point where he throws a tantrum. Imagine being 18 months old, and knowing what you want to do but not being able to do it for yourself or communicate clearly about it to someone else ... time and time again, every day. It would be enough to make any of us explode!

Setting limits

Being responsive as a parent needs to be balanced with an element of control to provide authoritative parenting. Parents need to be in charge in the family – healthy parenting does not mean that children always get their own way. Children feel secure if there are clear boundaries, which remain in place when they test them. The aim is to establish routines without rigidity, flexibility with some firmness. Consistency is an important component of positive parenting; without it, children become confused, insecure and often manipulative. An important part of growing up is learning to balance our own needs, desires and feelings with those of others. This is a gradual process, and a fine balancing act for parents. While very young children cannot be expected to see things clearly from another person's point of view, 11-year-olds who have not learnt that other people matter as much as they do can be hard to live with as they are usually so demanding.

Parents need to consider what routines and values are important to them, and then kindly to maintain and build on these. Some will be practical and domestic, such as always sitting down to have a drink rather than wandering around, or having a story and a cuddle at bedtime. Others are to do with treating others with respect, for example saying please and thank you, and waiting your turn to speak rather than interrupting when someone else is talking. Another category is what the family's leisure activities are and whether family members are fit and active or not, whether they take education seriously, or regularly attend church, temple, mosque or synagogue.

Many of us do not often reflect on our behaviours and attitudes – they are just part of who we are. Helping parents explore what is important to them may help to clarify the boundaries they will have with their children, and to examine whether these are fair and reasonable. Boundaries need to be like elastic: strong enough to stay in place, and yielding enough to expand as the child grows.

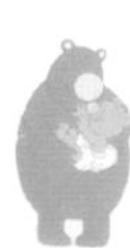

The behaviour that we expect from children needs also to be modelled by the adults around them. It is unfair to expect a child to stay seated during a meal if parents keep leaving the table; or not to make rude remarks if parents do so. Dramatic change can sometimes take place when parents recognise the importance of their own behaviour in shaping that of their children.

Discipline as guidance

Once limits have been set and boundaries are in place, children need discipline to help them learn to respect these. True discipline is not punishment, it is guidance: it helps a child to learn what is wanted, not to make them fear doing wrong. When we are critical of children or punish them we often tell them what they should not do but omit to tell them what we want instead. If a child is told, 'Don't look at me like that!' or 'You'll get a smack if you're naughty', he has learned only that the adult is angry; he is no clearer about how to behave. An alternative is to go to the other, indulgent extreme – never to correct a child for fear of being critical.

There is a middle way, which is another key feature of the HENRY approach to positive parenting: being clear about what we want by giving descriptive guidance. This is a winning combination with descriptive praise: one makes clear what we would like the child to do, the other recognises the child's co-operation and makes it easier for them to remember another time what is expected of them. (See below for more on praise.)

Here are some examples.

GUIDANCE AND PRAISE

Descriptive guidance	Descriptive praise
Please help me put the toys away in the box so they are safe.	Well done for putting the toys away in the box. I like it when we tidy up together.
I know you will share your toys nicely when your friends come to play.	I noticed how well you shared the toys; that was kind of you.
Be gentle with the cat, she likes to be stroked gently along her back, like this.	That's lovely. Listen, the cat is purring, she is happy when you stroke her gently.
It's teatime; let's sit down together.	I'm glad you enjoyed your tea; I did too.

Giving positive attention

Everyone needs attention, and babies and young children depend on it. Those who seem not to need it either receive so much that they can do without it for the brief time we are with them or – worryingly – have given up hope of receiving it.

Because attention is essential, children will get it in whatever way they can. Even being scolded or shouted at is better than nothing. A child who is ignored until he or she behaves badly, and only then is noticed, is unwittingly being trained to behave badly; a child who is given a lot of positive attention, and receives less attention for poor behaviour, is being trained to be more co-operative.

Positive attention both builds self-esteem and fosters positive behaviour. It includes sharing activities, enjoying each other's company, conversation, etc. and praise – the magic ingredient of positive attention.

Giving praise

Descriptive, genuine, warm, frequent praise from babyhood throughout childhood turns parents into self-esteem builders; frequent criticism turns us into demolition experts.

As the table above suggests, descriptive praise both acknowledges the behaviour that is being praised and reinforces it by being specific. It is easy to generalise when we praise, with phrases such as "What a good girl!" or "Brilliant!" While this is better than nothing, it does not make clear to the child just what it is they have done that has earned them the praise. In addition to being specific, praise needs to be genuine and to be given with a smile and a warm tone of voice.

Family rewards

Like praise, rewards help children to be clear about what behaviour is appreciated in the family. Rewards are different from bribery. A reward is an acknowledgement of co-operative behaviour, while a bribe is used to stop unwanted behaviour. The trouble with the latter is that it can reinforce the very behaviour we want to prevent. If a child runs off in the supermarket, and is told when the parent catches up with him, 'Now stop running off and I'll buy you a comic', what he learns is that running off gets him a comic. A reward, on the other hand, would be offered because the child stayed with the parent while they were shopping. Then the parent might say, 'You stayed with me as we agreed, so I'll buy you a comic.'

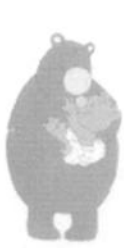

Many parents use food both to bribe and reward children, and also to offer comfort, or to show love. The food chosen is most often energy-dense 'treat' food such as ice cream or sweets. These foods acquire an emotional load that makes them seem particularly desirable. Using one food as a reward to encourage a child to eat another food (e.g. 'If you eat all your vegetables you can have your favourite chocolate pudding') is unhelpful for the same reason (see Chapter 5).

Rewards gain an extra value when they apply to all family members, not just to a young child. Rewards that anyone can earn, so that everyone is contributing to a family reward system, helps with consistency, feels fair, and fosters the idea that everyone in the family deserves to be recognised for keeping to the family's boundaries and routines, and treating each other well. In a collaborative family system, parents reward each other as well as their children, and children reward both each other and their parents. With young children, rewards need to be given frequently and the goal achieved in a short space of time, celebrated – and then another system introduced.

It is helpful to have a range of tokens for family rewards that cost little or nothing, appeal to children – and have nothing to do with food. Some examples are given below.

IDEAS FOR REWARDS FOR FAMILIES WITH YOUNG CHILDREN

- tokens to collect towards buying a family game
- a chart for coloured stickers or to colour in
- small items in a 'lucky dip' box
- a brick for a tower the family build to an agreed height
- reading an extra story together
- going on an outing

While this approach can feel strange at first, families who adopt it come to take pleasure in the positive atmosphere that results. A reward system encourages everyone to notice the family's strengths, rather than focusing most attention on any weaknesses, and can help with implementing new goals for the family – perhaps remembering to stay seated at mealtimes, trying new foods, or being more active together. Rewards particularly appeal to those who need visual as well as verbal reinforcement, and they lead to a sense of collective achievement. (Rewards given should never be taken away – whatever the behaviour was that merited the reward still stands.)

Giving children choices

It is worth considering how we feel when we experience a sense of powerlessness, and then to ask ourselves how often during the course of a day a young child may feel

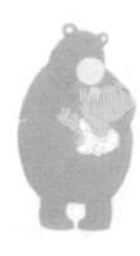

powerless. It can help us to understand a baby's screams and a toddler's tantrums rather better. We can also reflect on how overwhelming it can be when there are too many choices available.

It is helpful if – within the established boundaries – parents look for opportunities to empower their children by finding choices to give them. Attitudes to choice reflect parenting styles, as the chart below shows.

CHOICES FOR YOUNG CHILDREN

No choice (authoritarian)	Guided choice (authoritative)	Too much choice (indulgent)
Here's some carrot for your snack – eat it up.	Here are carrot and apple slices for your snack.	What would you like for your snack?
You're wearing these socks today.	Would you like to wear stripy socks or plain ones?	What do you want to wear today?
Off we go, we're walking to the park.	We're off to the park. Are you going to walk or ride your scooter?	What do you want to do this afternoon?
Make sure you eat what's in your lunchbox.	Would you like an egg or cheese sandwich in your lunchbox?	What shall I put in your lunchbox today?
It's bedtime. I'm going to read you this story now.	It's nearly time for your bedtime story. Would you like to choose it or shall I?	Do you feel like going to bed now?

When offering guided choices (the authoritative approach) the parent stays in charge by selecting alternatives that are suitable for the child's wellbeing, their age and stage of development, and are also manageable for the parent. An either–or choice is enough for a young child; as they mature, of course, a wider range of choices becomes appropriate.

It may take more thinking about, but reducing a young child's frustration is worth the effort, and giving them simple choices lays the foundations for responsible decision-making later in life.

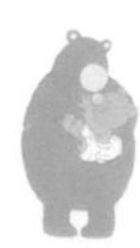

Enjoyment

Children need our company. This is as true of babies as it is of toddlers and older children. Some parents are comfortable chatting to their baby as they go about daily life. Others may be quite silent, either because it does not occur to them to talk to someone who can't yet speak, or because they feel foolish – or perhaps because they are feeling troubled and are unable to focus on the child's needs. A child's language development is influenced by how much they hear in their early months and years, so encouraging parents to converse has a long-term benefit as well as fostering a close relationship.

Sometimes the notion of parenting can become so serious. Children are happy when we enjoy their company, and the time we spend with them is so much more rewarding if we are enthusiastic and have fun together. In families where there is a great deal of pleasure, warmth and humour, there are likely to be children who are co-operative and positive; how much harder it is for them and for their parents when enjoyment is lacking. And how hard it can be for parents who are living in poverty, or are troubled, exhausted or unsafe, to enjoy their children.

As well as companionship, young children need us to engage in activities with them. It is important that some of these activities are energetic and promote physical development; these are explored in Chapter 7.

Key ideas

- parents' as well as children's needs are important
- realistic expectations give parents a helpful framework
- empathy is the cornerstone of responsive parenting
- setting clear, reasonable limits keep parents in charge
- the discipline children need is guidance, not punishment
- positive attention promotes positive behaviour
- helpful parenting strategies include: setting limits, descriptive guidance and praise, family rewards and giving children choices
- families need fun

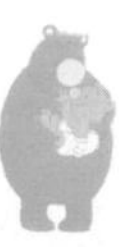

Exploring the issues with parents

How can we work with families to help promote the sort of parenting that will be conducive to a healthy lifestyle and emotional well-being?

The first thing to remember is that almost everyone is vulnerable in relation to their parenting. We all want to do the best for our children, but we may not be certain about just what 'best' is. In the same way that it is helpful for parents to be positive, empathic and appreciative with their children, so we need to be positive, empathic and appreciative of parents. As part of the relationship-building and exploring stages in the helping process (see Chapter 2) we need to seek opportunities to help parents recognise what is going well in the family, to highlight and praise their strengths. Emphasising the positive aspects of their parenting not only helps to build rapport between the parent and the helper, but also builds a parent's confidence.

Some parents will feel comfortable in their parenting role and yet may have lifestyle issues that it would be helpful for them to address. It is important not to assume that all parents are troubled about their parenting!

At the same time, we need to bear in mind that some people may not have encountered positive attitudes before in relation to the role of parents, either when they were children or as adults. Those who had an authoritarian or a neglectful childhood will bring these experiences into their adult lives, and into their parenting. Being encouraged to acknowledge their strengths, to accept praise for themselves or to be more responsive towards their own children, can sometimes feel strange and uncomfortable – and even plain wrong – if these attitudes are radically different from the parents' long-held views on how people are treated.

Parents who tend towards an indulgent style in their parenting may at first experience some difficulty with the idea that it is appropriate for them to take charge of the family, and to distinguish between a child's needs and their wants. These parents may be reacting against an authoritarian upbringing, and perceive the exercise of any control as repeating painful experiences that they are determined not to inflict on their own children. Some parents may not want to risk their child's disfavour, or may want to avoid any conflict and placate the child rather than consistently maintaining boundaries that have been set.

It is particularly important to recognise the context in which parents look after their children, because if we want to influence their parenting we may need to help them identify and challenge some of these echoes from the past, or some entrenched cultural attitudes. For example, if we observe that a mother's interaction with her child is characteristically withdrawn, it may be possible to help the mother become a more

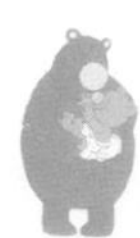

responsive parent only if we are first sensitive towards her needs, and can help her address the factors that are making her withdrawn (such as postnatal depression or loneliness). A father may also be disengaged when handling a baby, lacking confidence in his ability to meet the baby's needs. If parents are harsh disciplinarians, it is likely that parenting practices experienced in their own childhood or their community are being repeated, and gently encouraging them to review these will be helpful.

You will be able to gain some idea of the prevailing parenting style, and the quality of the relationship between the parent and child, just by observing their everyday interactions while you are with them. Is there physical closeness between them? What tone of voice does the parent use with the child – and the child with the parent? Is there more encouragement or more criticism? Do the parent's expectations of the child seem reasonable? Is the parent sensitive to the child's cues and needs? Do they enjoy each other's company in a warm and relaxed atmosphere, or is there anger or indifference? As well as forming a first impression, it is important to listen to the parent in order to find out whether what is going on is a typical pattern of behaviour or an exceptional one (for example, more difficult than usual because the child has been ill or the parent has a specific worry).

Your observations will be helpful in gaining a general idea of how the family may be functioning. It can be challenging for practitioners to remain emotionally open, and to maintain an empathic stance towards both parent and child, when the behaviour of either gives cause for concern. What is important is to encourage the parent to tell you how they feel about their relationship with the child, both in general and specifically around the question of food and healthy living. Remember that our aim is to explore and understand parents' own point of view, not just to help them gain awareness, confidence and skills.

Some parents feel anxious about their parenting and their relationship with the child generally. For others, anxiety is centred on food. While it can be tempting, within the context of tackling childhood obesity, to respond by focusing entirely on food, this is in practice seldom a helpful way forward in isolation from the broader issues in the parent–child relationship. At the same time, it is true that watching what happens during meals can offer a valuable springboard for discussion. The mealtime observation described in Chapter 5 may give you a good basis on which to explore more widely with parents how they feel about the relationship with their child as a whole, not just about food and mealtimes.

In a similar way, a parent who seeks advice because bedtime has become a battleground may initially want help to improve a child's behaviour. A more general exploration might reveal that the child would sleep better if they get more opportunities to be active during

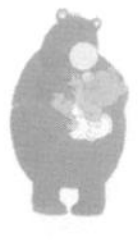

the day, or that bedtime has become a problem because the child is feeling insecure as a result of conflict between their parents – in other words, the apparent issue may have underlying causes that need to be addressed.

Whatever the immediate issue, taking time to consider together what aspects of parenting a parent feels happy with as well as what is not going so well, before moving on to what they would like to see improved (their goals), is likely to be time well spent. Once you have gained a fuller understanding of these issues, you can begin to explore how to achieve their goals by harnessing their strengths to seek solutions by extending what they already do and/or introducing new strategies to make family life run more smoothly.

Parenting programmes

A parent may be happy to experiment with new possibilities on their own and with your support, or they may be attracted to the idea of joining a group of parents interested in reflecting on and improving their parenting skills. These can be particularly useful for isolated parents because they widen a parent's social network as well as supporting them in their parenting role.

Until recently, the prevailing view was that parenting was something we all knew how to do, and suggesting that someone might benefit from help or advice was to suggest that they were inadequate. Fortunately, times are changing, and it is becoming more widely recognised that it is a sign of responsible parenting to seek new ideas about how to be a parent. There are websites, magazines and books devoted to the subject. The government supports the idea of universal parenting provision, and there are various effective group programmes – and training for those interested in facilitating groups – available in many parts of the country. It is worth finding out what is available in your area, for parents and for facilitators. HENRY also has a course for parents, which explores parenting support specifically within the context of healthy living and obesity prevention.

Endword

From the moment they are born, babies learn from every event and experience. Their developing brains are acutely finely tuned not only to their physical environment but also to the emotional atmosphere that surrounds them – in fact the brain is partly shaped by this. The early weeks, months and years of life have a significant impact on a person's capacity for healthy relationships, and at this time parents are a child's most important influence.

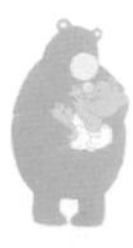

Parents also act as role models, and through our guidance and support have a major influence on every aspect of a child's life. Children learn from us even when we are not deliberately teaching them anything – and this includes our lifestyle.

Having explored the role of parenting and how we can support parents in developing more effective parenting skills, we will now examine more specifically how parenting relates to the key lifestyle areas of eating behaviour, nutrition and physical activity so essential to a healthy lifestyle.

References, further reading and resources

Baumrind D. Current patterns of parental authority. *Developmental Psychology Monographs* 1971, 4, 101–103

Dorman H & Dorman C. *The Social Toddler* Children's Project Publishing 2002

Gerhardt S. Why *Love Matters: How affection shapes a baby's brain* Brunner-Routledge 2004

Hunt C. *The Parenting Puzzle*: *How to Get the Best out of Family Life* Family Links 2003

Kelly G. *The Psychology of Personal Constructs* Norton 1955

Murray L & Andrews L *The Social Baby: Understanding babies' communication from birth* Children's Project Publishing 2000

Palmer S. *Toxic Childhood: How the modern world is damaging our children and what we can do about it* Orion 2006

Sunderland M. *The Science of Parenting* Dorling Kindersley 2006

Winnicott DW. *The Child, the Family and the Outside World*. Penguin 1964

Websites

Community Practitioners and Health Visitors Association (CPHVA) Parenting and Family Support Resources Bulletin
http://health.groups.yahoo.com/group/pafsinterestgroup

4

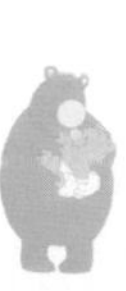

Family Links website
www.familylinks.org.uk

Parenting UK website
www.parentinguk.org

Let's Get Healthy with HENRY course for parents
http://www.henry.org.uk/training-courses.html#healthy

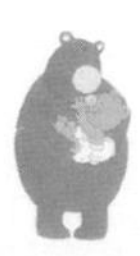

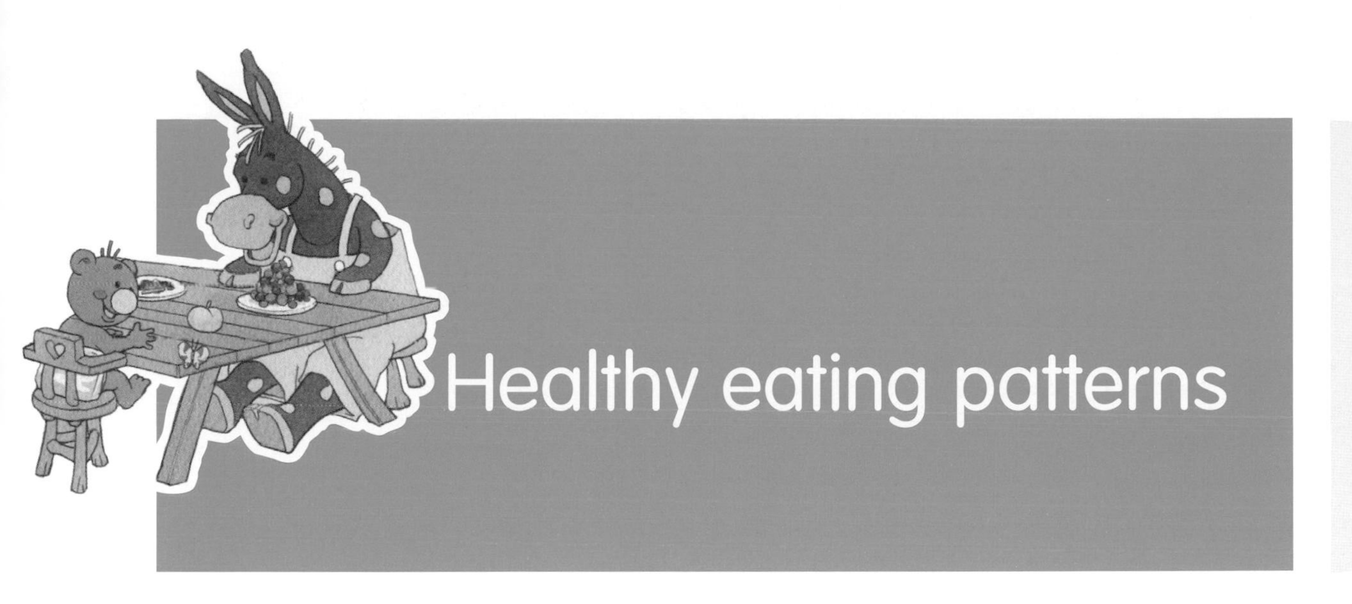

Healthy eating patterns

5

This chapter is central to working with families to promote a healthy lifestyle and prevent or reverse obesity. If we can help parents to establish healthy eating behaviour in their children, we will have gone a long way towards this. The issue of good eating habits is one that concerns parents and is therefore one that most will be open to explore, particularly if they have or know young children who are fussy about food.

In this chapter we will explore:

- the different influences at play in the development of children's eating behaviours
- children's hunger and fullness cues at different stages of development
- how to respect these cues and feed children responsively
- healthy patterns of eating
- how to gain an understanding of parents' attitudes to food, and the concerns they may have
- how to observe a mealtime and understand the parent–child interaction
- how to record a mealtime to explore this further
- useful strategies to help parents create a healthy eating environment for their children

Influences on the development of eating behaviour

If parents can set their children up to have a healthy approach to eating, there will be a less anxious focus on *what* they eat. Most parents find it stressful when children are faddy and demanding about food, so they are likely to appreciate support around mealtimes.

In order to work effectively in this area we need to understand what determines how we eat. There are four influences on our eating behaviour:

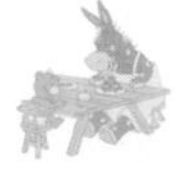

- hunger and appetite
- how we are taught to eat
- eating habits
- using food for non-nutritional reasons

Hunger and appetite

Hunger is the physical sensation caused by lack of food, whereas appetite is related to our enjoyment of food. Early on in life hunger is the main drive, but once babies are weaned, a healthy appetite needs to be fostered, along with an enjoyment of a wide range of foods.

Nowadays we rarely eat just to appease our hunger. It is nothing new to eat for social reasons, for comfort, because food tastes good and because we enjoy it. Our problem now is that food is so readily available and requires so little effort to prepare that we often overeat. For susceptible individuals, the result is excessive weight gain.

We are not born with an insatiable drive to eat. We know that babies (like any animal) have a finely tuned 'fuel gauge' that tells them when they need to eat and when they should stop. This information comes from research showing that if young babies are given high-energy milk they compensate by taking less. This compensation also occurs when breastfed babies are weaned – they cut back on the amount of milk they take.

So how is it that we lose the ability to eat sensibly and limit our eating to what our bodies need? It seems that this delicate fuel gauge is easily overridden by the way we are fed when we are young, and is influenced by the eating environment in which we grow up. This mattered little in the days when supplies of food were limited and we were very active. But nowadays children need to cope with an obesogenic environment, so it is particularly important to preserve their natural control mechanisms.

Most of the focus on obesity today is directed towards treating the already obese, or preventing its onset in older children who are already programmed to become obese. This chapter is about ensuring that young children preserve their ability to 'listen' to their bodies and so learn to eat only as much as they need. One important way to do this is to encourage parents to respect their baby's cues, and feed in a way that is responsive to their needs. Breastfeeding is a healthier option as, unlike bottle feeding, one can only breast-feed responsively. A mother cannot dictate what her baby takes, and in fact does not know how much has been taken. Her body is so in tune with the baby that she will only increase the amount of milk available in response to his needs. But breastfeeding is of course not enough to prevent obesity; many breast-fed children also cease to eat only when hungry by the time they are toddlers.

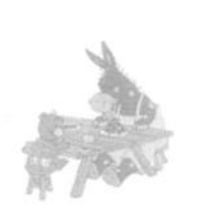

One key question is whether we are all born with a normal, healthy, and not excessive appetite. Might there be individuals whose fuel gauge is faulty and whose appetite is programmed to be either excessive or inadequate? There is no doubt that this does occur. We know, for example, that children born with hypothalamic conditions such as Prader Willi syndrome (see Chapter 8) develop an insatiable appetite as toddlers – their drive to eat dominates their existence. At the other end of the spectrum there are some babies with 'failure to thrive', who do not seem to experience an appropriate hunger drive and so fail to gain weight satisfactorily. However, most babies lie between these extremes and are born with an inherent ability to balance their food intake with their needs.

How we are taught to eat

Some interesting new work is emerging on how parents feed their children. Some children are urged to finish the food on their plates at every meal, sometimes with the threat of no dessert if they do not do so. In other families there is less insistence on eating everything that is provided. In yet others different food is prepared for each member of the family to make sure that everyone eats adequately, while in some households little attention is paid to the family's nutritional needs..

The four parenting styles described in Chapter 4 – authoritative, authoritarian, indulgent and neglectful – reflect how responsive a parent is towards their child's needs and how controlling they are of their child's behaviour. These styles have been extended to the context of feeding, and interestingly can be identified in families from very different cultures around the world. As with parenting generally, the preferred style is the authoritative style, in which the parent is responsive to the child's cues and needs, and at the same time stays in charge – in this context by offering healthy food choices, and setting clear boundaries. As with other aspects of parenting, when it comes to feeding, parents rarely fit neatly into a single category. They may use different styles on different days or with different children, or even within one meal. However, one approach generally predominates.

The concept of parenting styles is particularly important when working with obesity, as studies have shown that some feeding styles are linked to a child's later attitude to food and potentially to the development of obesity. For example, children whose parents have a predominantly authoritarian approach are more likely to be overweight. One can hypothesise that this may happen because an over-controlling parent decides exactly what and how much a young child should eat, with the danger that the child does not learn to respect their own cues. Likewise, when parents adopt a restrictive style and limit the amount and types of food eaten, or give certain foods only as a reward, their children also have an increased tendency to become overweight. This feeding style fosters a sense that the restricted food is excessively desirable – achieving the opposite effect to that

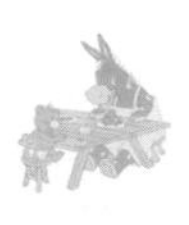

intended. At the other end of the spectrum, indulgent and neglectful feeding styles have also been linked with obesity.

The impact of these feeding styles is explored in more detail later in this chapter.

Eating habits

One of the tasks of parenting is to introduce structure into babies' lives, establishing a pattern of sleeping at night, eating at mealtimes, and so on. Structure is important. One of the reasons put forward for the obesity epidemic in the UK is our loss of family mealtimes. Many children (and adults) today snack whenever the mood takes them, and never experience the sensations of hunger and fullness. One reason why countries such as France have a lower rate of obesity may be that family mealtimes are still the norm.

It may appear paradoxical to say that children's feelings of hunger and fullness should be respected, and yet claim that structured mealtimes need to be established. There is in fact no paradox – balance is the key. The role of the parent is to provide nutritious food at regular intervals, while the child decides how much to eat. It is important that babies are fed responsively, and also that they are gradually weaned on to regular mealtimes.

Research suggests that children who have lost their innate sense of when they are hungry or full can be helped to relearn it. A fascinating study by Leann Birch and Susan Johnson in the United States illustrates this. They gave a group of pre-schoolers dolls with detachable stomachs filled with salt. Some of the stomachs were filled to bursting, some were half filled and some were left empty. The children were encouraged to attach onto their doll the stomach that most appropriately described their own sense of fullness after a snack. The researchers noted that children whose mothers were obese found it more difficult to select an appropriate stomach. Over time the children learnt to be sensitive to their feelings of fullness, and by the end of the study they chose to eat less at a meal if it was preceded by a high-energy snack. This work is encouraging as it suggests that children can learn to respect their internal cues about how much to eat.

Using food for non-nutritional reasons

One of the most fundamental aspects of parenting is providing food for our children, enjoying their contentment and watching them grow. It is no surprise that when a baby fails to thrive it is very distressing for parents. Food is symbolic of our love for our children, and has a central role in all cultures. The problem is that in our obesogenic environment we are harming our children by using food so readily and frequently as treats, rewards, comfort, relief of distress and to show our love. A cultural change is

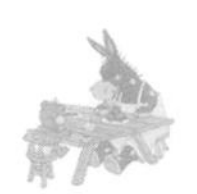

needed so that adults offer and value alternatives to food in these situations. This message needs to extend beyond the immediate family. Grandparents, child minders, nurseries and schools all need to be on board. Parents of our obese patients tell us how distressed and angry they are when sweets or chocolate are given as awards for achievement.

Key ideas

- Left to their own devices, most young children have a natural 'fuel gauge' that dictates how much they need to eat
- It is important for parents to be responsive to their child's cues
- Excessively controlling and restrictive feeding, as well as indulgent and neglectful feeding, are linked to obesity
- Structured family mealtimes generate healthier patterns of eating than frequent snacking or grazing through the day
- Using food to reward good behaviour, as treats and to comfort distressed children contributes unhelpfully to children's attitudes towards food

5

Creating a healthy eating environment

The key to creating a healthy family eating environment lies in establishing structure, with regular mealtimes where children learn to appreciate food in the company of others without distractions such as television. The first steps lie in helping parents to recognise their baby's hunger and fullness cues, and to feed them responsively.

Hunger and fullness cues

When parents respect babies' cues from the start, the babies themselves learn to appreciate their own sensations and are more likely to eat only as much as they need. When babies' feelings of fullness are overridden they are more likely to overeat even when they do not feel like it, and this can become a pattern that carries on in later life.

Newborn babies readily cry when hungry, and have a very clear sense of when they are full. There was a period not so long ago when babies were fed according to a schedule. We have now moved back to feeding them 'on demand'. On one level this is good as it

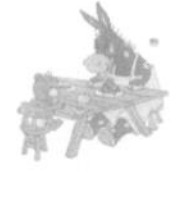

HUNGER AND FULLNESS CUES

	Newborn 0–4 mths	Head up 4–6 mths	Sitting 6–8 mths	Crawling 8–12 mths	Beginning to walk 12–15mth	Toddler 15–24 mths
SIGNS OF HUNGER	Cries or fusses Gazes at caregiver Opens mouth when ready to feed	Cries or fusses Smiles and gazes at carer during feeding	Cries or grizzles Leans forward towards spoon Reaches out to food Intent on feeding	Cries or grizzles Grabs spoon or food Points to food	May be irritable but this does not always mean hungry Asks for foods with sounds, words or gestures	Takes carer to cupboard or fridge to show what is wanted
SIGNS OF FULLNESS	Stops sucking Spits out nipple or falls asleep Arches back away	Spits out nipple or falls asleep Stops sucking Arches back away	Turns head away or arches away from spoon Easily distracted from eating Spits food back	Slows down in eating Clenches mouth shut or pushes food away Easily distracted from eating	Shakes head to say "no more" Plays with food rather than eating it Plays with food rather than eating it	Uses words like "all done" and "get down" Plays with food or drops it to floor
HELPFUL TIPS	Let baby decide how much to take – there's no need to finish the bottle If baby cries and has fed recently, try to comfort without milk – not all crying is hunger	Let baby decide how much to take – still no need to finish the bottle! If baby cries and has fed recently, try to comfort without milk – not all crying is hunger Solid foods are not yet needed	If baby wakes at night check nappy, offer brief cuddle or water – try not to give milk Let baby to touch food	Encourage finger foods and let baby have a spoon too Give small portions Let baby enjoy handling food even if it makes a mess Begin to have set mealtimes and snacktimes Try not to feed baby at night	Encourage finger foods and let baby use a spoon Give small portions Let baby enjoy handling food even if it makes a mess Begin to have set meal times and snacktimes Try not to give baby a bottle	Encourage child to eat independently rather than be fed Try to eat together as a family Continue to discourage grazing Comfort or reward child with something other than food

encourages parents to be responsive to their babies' needs, but there is a danger in it – any cry may be assumed to be one of hunger. The baby is then not only overfed, but can also learn that all distress is best alleviated with food. While it would not be desirable to return to the rigid schedule of feeding imposed in the 1950s, it is important that parents try to understand their baby's distressed cry for what it is, rather than assuming that feeding is always required, particularly if it is not long since the last feed.

As babies develop, the way they express their feelings of hunger and fullness changes. The chart shows how these cues change from the newborn period to the age of two years,

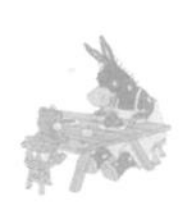

beyond which children are usually able to say if they are hungry or full. The chart also provides some helpful hints for parents at different stages.

Authoritative feeding and how to achieve it

In the previous section we explored different styles of feeding, the ways these may affect how a young child eats and their influence on the likelihood of the child later becoming obese. The ideal feeding style is authoritative: the parent is sensitive and responsive to the child's hunger and fullness cues in a warm, nurturing and structured environment, participation is encouraged and yet appropriate limits are set for what type of food is eaten, and behaviour that is suitable for mealtimes (that depends on the age of the child).

The first step in moving towards more authoritative feeding is for a parent to understand their baby's or child's cues and to respond appropriately. At the same time the parent needs to make mealtimes an enjoyable social experience.

There are seven steps to achieving this:

Setting
The mealtime needs to be structured, with parent and child sitting down together away from distractions such as television and toys, and a consistent feeding/mealtime schedule.

Positioning
The best position for feeding is for the parent to sit opposite the baby so that it is easy to relate, to see the baby's expression and use a spoon. Later on, when the toddler is eating independently, this position may change but it should still encourage sociable mealtimes.

Mood and atmosphere
An important aim is to make mealtimes enjoyable, rather than simply a time for eating. This is perhaps even more important than focusing on what the child actually eats. Both the parent's and the child's mood contribute to the mealtime atmosphere. If parents appreciate that this is important they can put some thought into making it positive and pleasant.

Participation
Both parent and child need to take part in the mealtime. This should happen from babyhood and continue through to independent eating. One important parenting goal is to foster this independence. To do so parents need to have a clear idea about when they can expect their baby to begin to finger feed, drink from a cup, manage a spoon and eventually wield a fork and knife.

Pacing
The rhythm for the meal needs to be set by the baby. There should be a pause for swallowing and taking a breath between each mouthful; there is a tendency to overfeed if another spoonful is introduced before the previous mouthful is finished. The rhythm of a meal can be disrupted when parents become concerned that their baby or toddler has not eaten enough. On the other hand, extending mealtimes excessively (beyond 20 minutes or so) is rarely helpful.

Encouragement
Encouragement is not the same as pressure. It is often counterproductive if there is excessive focus on what the child eats, though young children may need gentle encouragement to try new foods, and to develop their eating skills. Parents often find the messy stage of learning to eat trying; a focus on social eating is easier once children can proudly feed themselves.

Conversation
An important feature of a mealtime is communication. Some parents may need encouragement to initiate a conversation with their baby. Talking encourages a close bond between parent and child, as well as eating and language skills. Perhaps the biggest bar to this is television, as it is distracting and makes communication difficult.

Unhelpful feeding styles

If our goal is to promote authoritative feeding, in what ways are other feeding styles unhelpful? When supporting parents it can be helpful for us to be aware of the characteristics of each style so we can help them move towards being more consistently authoritative.

It is important to emphasise that the descriptions given below are caricatures designed to give us a way of thinking about different styles for feeding babies and young children. It is unhelpful to typecast parents into any one style. The aim is to have a framework that can help us explore issues with parents and encourage them to be both responsive to their child and able confidently to establish boundaries for eating and mealtime behaviour (the authoritative style already described).

The authoritarian style
In this style parents try to control everything during a feed or meal, including what, how much, and the pace and manner in which food is eaten. If they decide that the child has not eaten enough they make the child eat more. Instead of encouraging the child to finger feed or hold a spoon, they may keep a tight grip on the spoon so that they have full control and prevent the child from exploring their food or trying to feed themselves. It

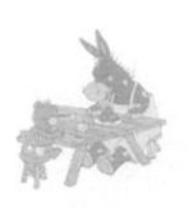

may not take long for the child to lose respect for their own appetite and eat more than necessary. Mealtimes may also become a battleground as the child pits his will against that of the parent.

A restricting style is also authoritarian, reflecting the parent's concern that the child may eat more than is healthy or that they will eat the wrong sort of foods. Parents may remove food before the child has finished, refuse to allow second helpings or prevent the child from eating certain foods. The problem is that the child is likely to develop a strong desire for the forbidden foods and eat these whenever they can.

The indulgent style
In this style, parents are sensitive and responsive to their child's hunger and fullness cues, but give in to every whim – they meet the child's wants rather than their needs. This is not healthy because not everything a child wants is necessarily best for him or her. Another reason is that all children need boundaries in order to feel secure.

The neglectful style
In this style, parents pay little attention to the child or to what they are eating. There is a lack of interest in children and their nutritional needs, and once the child has independent access to food they may well overeat.

Healthy patterns of eating

The healthiest eating behaviour involves structured mealtimes. It is difficult to turn our culture around now, but there is no doubt that one key to healthy living and reducing obesity is promoting change in family eating patterns.

Three plus two
Some parents may find it hard to recognise when babies no longer need to be fed on demand and are ready to be moved towards having structured mealtimes with the family. As a result, young children learn to 'graze' through the day rather than settling down to a regular pattern of mealtimes where they are more likely to respond appropriately to their hunger and fullness cues.

The recommendation to eat three meals and two snacks a day is especially important in the childhood years. To encourage healthy eating it is helpful to consider that the snack times are mini-meals, and that all food and drink is eaten as a meal, with a clear beginning and end, rather than being eaten while playing or on the move. The quality of the snacks is also important as so many snacks contain more calories than children nutritionally need.

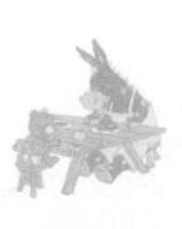

EATING PATTERNS TO AIM FOR

- 3 meals a day
- 2 sit-down snack times
- family mealtimes
- discourage grazing

The three Ss

The three Ss are a helpful concept to encourage a healthy pattern of eating. Many people put on excess weight because of what they eat between meals rather than at meals. The three Ss remind us that food is best eaten:

- sitting down
- slowly
- sociably

Adopting this approach helps us develop a more mindful attitude to how we eat, respect for hunger and fullness cues and enjoyable mealtimes.

Family mealtimes

Many families do not eat round a table, but this need not be a barrier to sociable mealtimes. It is not our remit to recommend how a family should eat, but it is helpful to encourage a family lifestyle that has a sociable approach to food. It is helpful for parents to know that setting aside the time to eat together, and to enjoy each other's company while doing so, will help young children achieve a healthier approach to food.

Television

Television needs special consideration as it is such a hindrance to sociable eating, as well as having a strong negative effect on children's activity levels (see Chapter 7). When the television is on during meals, viewers can become so absorbed in watching that they are unaware of what they are eating and become oblivious of any signs of fullness. It also has an effect on social aspects of eating, getting in the way of family members talking together at mealtimes.

Television is particularly insidious as an activity for anyone in the family, as unlike most other activities (even computer games), it is so often accompanied by snacking. More often than not, the food eaten is energy dense, and so imposes the double effect of minimal expenditure of energy with significant intake.

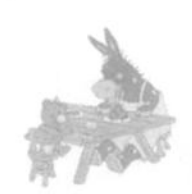

Another important aspect to consider in relation to television and young children is advertising. Until children are at least 7 years old they do not understand that advertising is designed to influence them. They believe the messages to be the truth, and are therefore particularly susceptible to the power of the media. The food industry fully appreciates this vulnerability, and plays on the power of young children to pester their parents to buy particular products. Parents need to be aware of this so they set limits not only on the amount of time their children spend watching television but also what they watch, and have the confidence to resist their children's pleas.

Key ideas

- Hunger and fullness cues need to be respected
- The ideal feeding style is authoritative, where the parent is responsive and also sets and maintains boundaries
- Positioning, atmosphere, communication, encouragement, rhythm and participation are important components in feeding young children
- A healthy eating pattern is to eat '3+2' meals/snacks a day
- Eating according to the 3 Ss – sitting down, slowly and sociably – is a helpful approach
- Family mealtimes can promote healthy eating
- Television has a negative effect by blocking fullness cues and conversation, and because of the influence of advertising

Exploring the issues with parents

Establishing and maintaining healthy eating patterns can be a real challenge for parents, especially when others around them pay no attention to this. Yet it is key to tackling and preventing obesity. It is an area that particularly benefits from the HENRY approach, as sensitivity is needed to explore attitudes and concerns. When parents have concerns, you may at times find it helpful to suggest that you observe a mealtime. It will help you understand what is going and make it easier to support the parents in finding ways to make mealtimes easier for them and for their child.

Exploring concerns, behaviour and attitudes to eating

Eating behaviour is a concern in many families and often becomes significant when a child is overweight or obese. In looking at a child's eating behaviour it is worth remembering that we are in effect examining that of the parent as well – and parents are aware of this. Some parents may be quite defensive towards health professionals, particularly when they have previously felt judged.

In addition to building a trusting relationship with parents, taking a solution-focused approach in which you invite a parent to explore with you everything that is going well in the family around mealtimes and eating behaviour will help to dissolve their discomfort. Rather than looking for parents' weaknesses, highlight their strengths through your interest and encouragement, and then build on these. When you have come to a common understanding of eating patterns and attitudes to food in the family as a whole, you will be able to begin to help them set goals that address their concerns, and plan how to achieve these.

The exploration process will of course depend on the age of the child, and whether parents think there are problems around feeding or weight gain. Even if there are not, parents are likely to have views about young children's eating, and experience of difficulties that friends or relatives have had around food.

Particular issues that it may be valuable to explore include:

- Does the young child have set mealtimes or does he tend to 'graze' through the day?
- How good an appetite does the child have?
- How independently does the child eat and is this appropriate for their age?
- Does the child feel satisfied after a meal or does he constantly ask for more?
- Are there concerns around eating, for this or any other child? If so, what does the parent think may be the cause?
- How does this affect the rest of the family, and what have the parents tried so far?
- Is food used for rewards or treats?
- Does the family usually eat together (round a table if culturally appropriate) or are mealtimes for children separate from those of adults?
- Does the family eat with the television off or on?
- At what age do the children have independent access to food?
- Are there family members such as grandparents or a childminder who have an influence on the children's eating?

In exploring these issues the art lies in eliciting information by encouraging the parent to talk, not by asking a barrage of questions. The exploration will be most successful if you

listen attentively to the parent's views and feelings. This may be all that is needed to enable you and the parent to understand the situation well enough. If so, you will then move on to thinking about what the parent would like to change and how to go about this. On the other hand, it may be helpful to explore further by arranging to observe a meal or even go on to record a mealtime on video or DVD that you can use as a basis for discussion.

Observing a meal

We can learn much by simply talking through parents' feelings and views about their child's eating, and exploring how the family eats. We can sometimes help them by discussing what they know about influences on children's eating patterns and how to establish a healthy eating environment. However, when there are still concerns about a child's eating (whether over- or under-eating) there is no substitute for actually observing a mealtime. This is an important aspect of the HENRY approach and we have compiled a DVD to help practitioners develop this skill.

When you observe a meal you can learn more about:

- how a child signals hunger and fullness – and how the parent responds
- how independently the child eats
- the parent's feeding style and strategies
- the mood of the meal
- what a child eats

Health professionals are often cautious about suggesting that they watch a meal, but in our experience parents usually welcome the suggestion and feel reassured that their concerns will be better understood. You may need to explain that the purpose is to share thoughts about what you have seen and use this as a basis for moving forwards, not to be critical.

Start by asking the parent where they normally sit and where would be the best place for you. You want to make sure you can see the interaction between the child and parent without influencing it. Ask the parent to tell you when the meal is starting and when it is finished. It is very important not to comment or intervene during the meal, as this could change what takes place.

You need to have a framework for observing the meal. We favour one that allows you to look for how responsive the feeding process is, to identify any unhelpful feeding approaches and to observe the foods that are provided. An outline of the principles is shown below.

TUNING IN TO MEALTIMES

Look out for the following:

Helpful approaches

- *Setting* Is the parent sitting down with the child, and setting appropriate boundaries away from other distractions?
- *Positioning* Are the parent and child positioned well (face to face) to allow for good communication?
- *Mood and atmosphere* Is the mealtime pleasant and affectionate?
- *Participation* How much does the child take part in the feeding process? If the child is old enough, is independence in eating encouraged?
- *Pacing* The rhythm should be led by the child's own hunger and fullness cues, and monitored by the parent to ensure that food is eaten at a moderate pace. Is the parent attentive to the cues being given? (see [table 5.1])
- *Encouragement* Does the parent calmly and gently encourage the child to eat?
- *Conversation* Are parent and child communicating comfortably?

Unhelpful approaches

- *Over-encouragement* Pleading, bribes, commands, distractions, and direct attempts to get the food in despite signals that the child does not want to eat. Although the intentions are usually positive, the effect is negative as the child either becomes more resistant or is led to overeat; mealtimes become more stressful.
- *Under-encouragement* Is the child eating alone, is the parent distracted, negative or not an active participant? Is television a distraction?
- *Indulgence* Does the parent allow the child to play excessively with the food, or give the child whatever he or she wants if the child is picky or demanding?

Food offered (see Chapter 6)

- *Types of food* What food is provided?
- *Balance* How balanced is the meal?
- *Texture* Is it appropriate for the child's age?
- *Portion size* Is an appropriate amount of food offered?

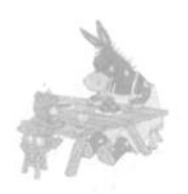

Recording a meal

You and the parents may wish to explore mealtimes further by recording a mealtime. The additional value of this is that you can share the recording with the parent and reflect together on how the child is eating and what might be changed to encourage a healthier approach to food. If necessary, it also allows you (with the parent's permission) to show the recording to experienced colleagues and obtain their advice about a way forward.

You need to discuss the idea with the parent when you have explored the issues around eating. Reassure them that the purpose is for you to look at the recording together and learn from it. If they agree, then suggest that you do it at the next visit. It is a good idea to ask them to sign a consent form, so that you can keep the recording and review it later.

The principles when recording a mealtime are the same as for a straightforward observation. Set up the camera so that you can see the interactions between child and parent. Ask to be told when the meal starts and when it is finished. Once again, it is important that you do not comment or intervene during the meal.

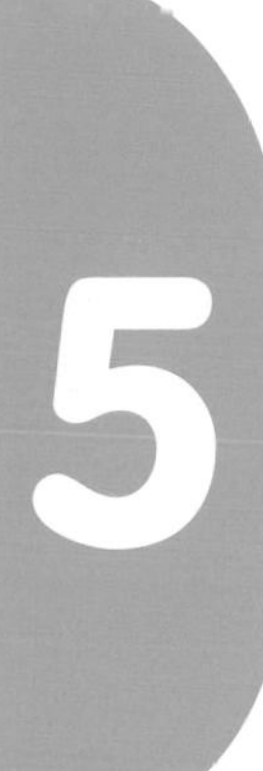

Sharing feedback

Whether you have observed a meal or recorded it, the time spent afterwards sharing feedback can be valuable. It is all too easy to leap in with well-intentioned criticism and advice, rather than encouraging the parent's own observations, supporting their views and insight, and adding your own as sparingly as possible. The steps for ensuring that feedback is a positive and genuinely joint process are outlined below.

It is always best to ensure that you both look for the positive features first, rather than highlighting problems. (It is quite likely that the parent will be more negative than you are.) Asking whether the mealtime was a typical one will help you avoid the trap of forming opinions about a meal that does not reflect the child's usual eating behaviour. Encouraging the parent to feed back first is respectful, and can also make giving your feedback easier as you may well find that their observations pre-empt your own, so all you will need to do is acknowledge what the parent has noticed.

When you give your feedback, use your encouraging comments to highlight the importance of responsive feeding, and emphasise ways in which the parent already demonstrates this. When the time comes to mention less helpful tactics, make sure you explore the reasons for these rather than simply criticising or correcting the parent's behaviour. You might say, 'I noticed that you held Sam's hands while you fed him. I wonder what the reason for this was?' rather than 'It isn't a good idea to hold your child's hands while you are feeding him'.

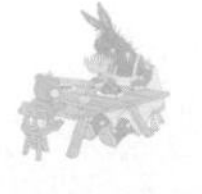

SHARING FEEDBACK

There are 7 steps in sharing feedback.

1 Offer a positive comment about the meal you have just observed – be specific and descriptive in your praise.
2 Ask the parent for their view, encouraging them also to focus on what went well; check whether the meal was typical of how the child usually eats
3 Explore what the parent thought did not go so well, and why
4 Offer your feedback, again starting with the positive, and taking into account what the parent has already mentioned
5 Move on to explore together what might be improved, again seeking the parent's ideas
6 Draw together your joint conclusions
7 Decide together on what changes the parent thinks may be helpful, ending on a positive note

When both of you have fed back your thoughts, summarising the discussion will maintain a clear focus; again, it is important to involve the parent in the process – perhaps, for example, by asking them what they think the most important points are. The parent may want time to reflect, or may be ready to think about some goals and develop an action plan.

If you have recorded a meal you may find it better to watch it and go through the feedback process at a separate visit. This will give you time to view the recording yourself in advance, though there then is a danger of your being more familiar with the recording than the parent and reverting to advice-giving rather than strengths-based support. When you sit down with the parent, watch the recording all the way through; if the parent is comfortable, you could suggest that you both jot down your thoughts. (When a parent does not want to do this, it is better if you don't do it either.) Then move on to sharing back together – you may want to review sections as you do so. Some parents can become upset when watching or reviewing the recording, particularly if they realise that they persisted in feeding when the child gave clear cues that they had had enough. Self-awareness can be a painful process, so you need to offer particularly sensitive and empathic support.

When you have completed the feedback process, it is good to remember to ask the parent what they would like to happen to the recording. They often wish to keep it.

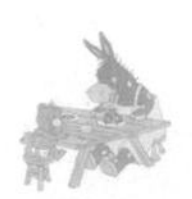

Endword

Adopting a healthy eating pattern is a vital component in leading a healthy lifestyle. If we can help parents feed babies responsively and establish healthy eating behaviour for the family, we will have gone a long way towards this goal. In this chapter we have looked at the various influences at play in the development of children's eating behaviours, before moving on to practical strategies that will help children develop a pattern of healthy eating – one that can stand them in good stead for life.

In the next chapter we will consider what children eat and how we can help families to eat more healthily. Introducing young children to a healthy nutritional diet from the start helps to ensure that they will eat more healthily throughout their lives.

References, further reading and resources

Dietz W. Eating behaviors of the young child in *Eating Behaviours of the Young Child – prenatal and postnatal influences on healthy eating* Eds Birch L & Dietz W. American Academy of Pediatrics 2008

Faith MS. Scanlon KS et al. Parent-child feeding strategies and their relationships to child eating and weight status. Obesity Research 2004; 12: :1711–22.

Fisher JO and Birch LL. Restricting access to palatable foods affects children's behavioural; response, food selection and intake. *American Journal of Clinical Nutrition* 1999; 32:405–419

Fomon SJ. *Nutrition of Normal Infants* St Louis, MP: Mosby-Yearbook; 1993

Fomon SJ, Filmer LJ et al. Influence of formula concentration on caloric intake and growth of normal infants. *Acta Paediatrica Scandinavica* 1975; 64:172–181

Fox MK, Devaney B, Reidy K. Razafindrakoto C, Ziegler P. Relationship between portion size and energy intake among infants and toddlers: evidence of self-regulation *J Am Diet Assoc* 2006 Jan; 1061 (1 Suppl 1):S77–83

Johnson SL and Birch LL . Parents and children's adiposity and eating style. *Pediatrics* 1994; 94:653–661

Johnson SL Improving Preschoolers' Self Regulation of Energy Intake. *Pediatrics* 2000 106: 1429–1435

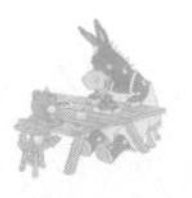

Patrick H, Nicklas TA. The benefits of authoritative feeding style: parent feeding styles and children's food consumption patterns. *Appetite* 2005; 44:243–249

Rhee KE, Lumen JC et al. Parenting styles and overweight status in first grade. *Pediatrics* 2006; 117:2047–2054

Savage JS, Fisher JO and Birch LL. Parental influence on eating behavior: conception to adolescence. *Journal of Law, Medicine & Ethics* 2007; 35(1):22–34,

Vandewater EA. Linking TV viewing and children's obesity in *Eating Behaviours of the Young Child – prenatal and postnatal influences on healthy eating* Eds Birch L & Dietz W. American Academy of Pediatrics 2008 pp 101–122

DVDs and videos

Tuning in to Mealtimes: Helping parents and carers develop responsive feeding
Mary Rudolf and Candida Hunt
www.henry.org.uk

Baby-led weaning
Gill Rapley
sales@markittelevision.com

Clues from Children's Mealtimes: a video and teaching manual on eating difficulties in young children
Pauline Raynor and Mary Rudolf
Media services, University of Leeds
mediaservices@leeds.ac.uk

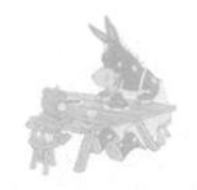

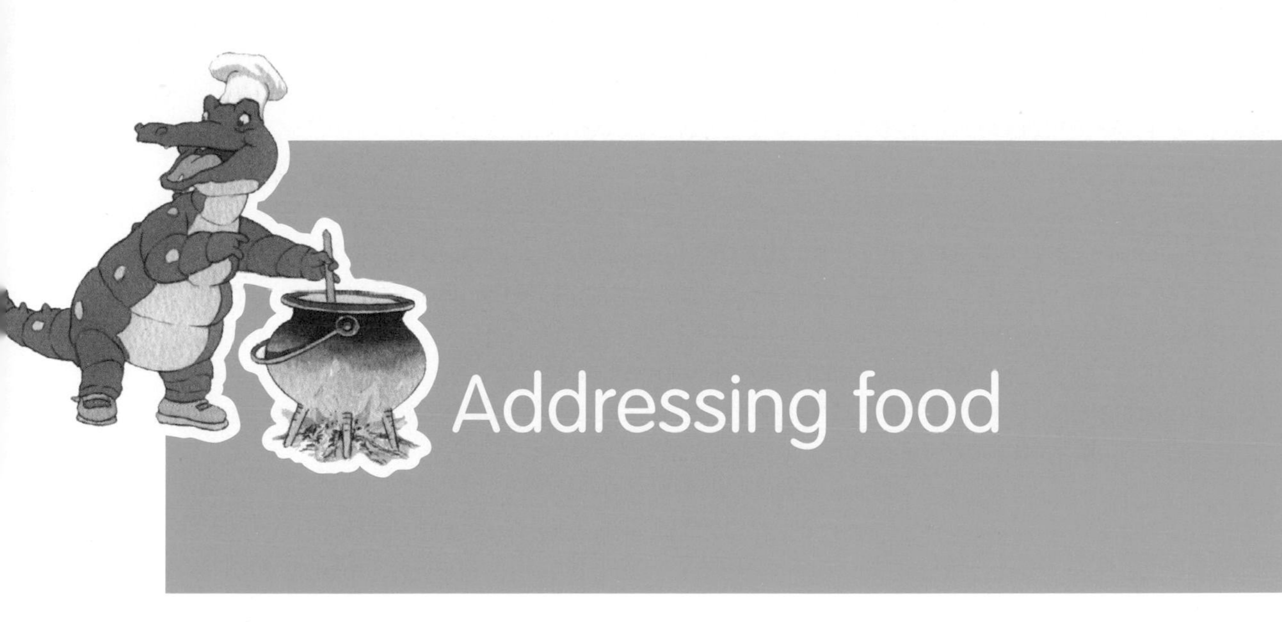

Addressing food

6

Food is one of the principal ways that we nurture our children, and a source of both delight and anxiety. As a healthy diet in the early years lays the foundations for good nutrition throughout life, we can make a real contribution through the support we give families at this time. Many parents seek guidance, and are willing to examine their family's eating habits so that their infant has a healthy start. This gives an opportunity for informal discussions about food and health, and for us to offer positive messages about good eating habits.

In this chapter we will explore:

- how parents shape their children's diet and the food they eat
- the constituents of a healthy balanced diet and appropriate portion sizes
- how to encourage parents to optimise infant feeding in the first six months
- how to support parents through the stages of weaning
- how to help the baby or young child who has unhealthy weight gain
- how to gain a clear picture of what the baby/young child is eating
- useful strategies to help parents encourage their children to eat healthily

What influences the food children eat?

The most powerful influence on what children eat comes from their parents, whose beliefs and knowledge determine what food is offered. They also affect what their child eats by how they model and shape mealtimes, and by deciding the sort of foods to keep in the home. Other carers, whether these are family members such as grandparents, a childminder or nursery staff, can have a strong influence too, as can the food provided in childcare settings.

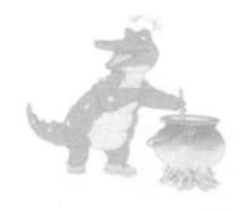

Parents' beliefs and knowledge

We all have certain beliefs about food based on our previous experience both in childhood and as adults. Family, social and cultural norms are strong. Some parents are traditional in their attitudes to food, while others are more open to new ideas about healthy eating, are keen to acquire nutrition knowledge, and are concerned about the possible risk of their child being overweight. Different family members are likely to have different beliefs and expectations, which may be confusing or lead to outright conflict.

Nutrition knowledge appears to play a small though pivotal part in the adoption of healthier food habits. Parents' nutrition knowledge is positively related to healthier eating, so it is important that parents have access to accurate information. There is considerable misunderstanding regarding current healthy eating guidelines. Those based on the Food Standards Agency's Eatwell plate food groups promote variety, balance and moderation. Nevertheless, there is a widespread view that there are 'good' or 'bad' foods, and those that are unhealthy in large amounts (such as sugar) are also harmful in small amounts. This misunderstanding leads to an over-emphasis on 'good' foods and restriction of 'bad' foods, which may give rise to inappropriate feeding practices that result in a child acquiring strong preferences for the restricted foods and a dislike of the food that is promoted.

It is clear that in addition to nutrition knowledge, parents' beliefs and preferences greatly influence their attitudes to food – as do our own. It is important to understand these if we are to help the families we support.

Modelling

Parents are influential role models for their children when it comes to food just as they are in other areas of family life. For example, research shows similarities in many aspects of mothers' and daughters' intake, including what they drink, their consumption of fruit and vegetables, and their fat, mineral and vitamin intake. These findings may reflect a number of factors such as the types of foods that the mother prefers and consequently offers the child; the exposure to and accessibility of these foods within the home, and the opportunity for children to eat together with adults at mealtimes.

Many people have double standards, expecting children to eat certain foods that are good for them despite disliking – and therefore not eating – the food themselves. In order to learn to enjoy a wide range of healthy foods, children need to see their parents doing so. One of the strongest influences on a child's willingness to try new foods is to witness their parents eating, particularly if the parents are clearly enjoying the experience. This is why we promote sociable eating so strongly. It is a strange development in recent years

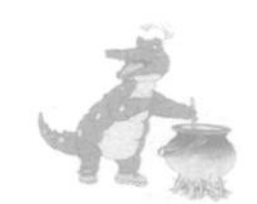

that children are so often expected to eat child-specific foods such as fish fingers and chicken nuggets, rather than participating in a family meal where all members of the family eat the same food. This has no doubt been influenced by the food industry, which has succeeded in shaping children's eating preferences.

Shaping

Parents and other carers are influential in moulding children's eating habits in other ways, too. One is by using foods as rewards or for comfort (see Chapter 4). One of the strategies often used is to restrict foods considered to be bad and encourage foods considered to be good. The preferred food may be used as a reward for eating the less preferred food – for example, 'If you eat your vegetables then you can have your dessert'.

Such strategies are counter-productive as they add emotional value to the 'reward' food, encouraging a preference for it. Buying but then restricting access to sweets, crisp-type snacks and biscuits actually increases the preference for and consumption of these foods even when restrictions are no longer imposed. This has been linked to increased eating in the absence of hunger in girls and an increased intake of fat.

Instructing a child to 'eat up' or 'clear your plate' is also unhelpful. What we need is to know what size portions are appropriate for children at different ages (see below), and to respect their hunger and fullness cues (see Chapter 5).

Flavours and food preferences

What we eat is also determined by our very earliest feeding experiences. Our food preferences have their roots way back into babyhood – even the way we were fed as infants has an influence. Babies' likes and dislikes for different flavours can be shaped in the early weeks and even before they are born.

This is illustrated by some fascinating studies carried out by Dr Julie Mennella in the United States. She knew that farmers give pregnant sows the food they will later want the piglets to eat to improve their growth, and decided to see if this was true for babies too. She recruited women during pregnancy, and asked one group to drink carrot juice towards the end of the pregnancy but not when breastfeeding. The second group were asked to drink carrot juice when they were breastfeeding but not during pregnancy, and the third to avoid carrots and carrot juice altogether.

When the babies were ready for weaning they were all given rice cereal mixed with carrot juice, and mothers and researchers recorded the effect. Dr Mennella found that the babies

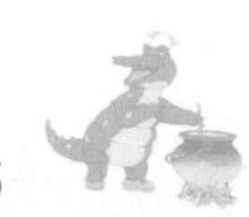

whose mothers had drunk carrot juice when pregnant or breastfeeding accepted the cereal readily, but the others did not! The message is clear – babies like to eat what their mothers eat in pregnancy and during lactation. This makes good sense. If young animals come across flavours they met during pregnancy or in their mother's milk, they can be confident that the food is safe to eat. A *new* flavour is probably best avoided, as it might be dangerous.

Other research has shown that the flavours we meet in infancy have an effect beyond those early months. Researchers have studied babies born with a condition called PKU, who cannot drink ordinary breast or formula milk and need to have a very unpleasant 'elemental' formula instead. When these babies were followed up years later as teenagers, they were quite prepared to drink the formula (even though they had not had it since they were babies), whereas their friends rejected it out of hand. This supports other research that tells us that what we eat as babies has an influence on what we like to eat later, and emphasises the importance of making sure that children learn to eat healthily from the start.

Accessibility

An important starting point for ensuring that children eat healthily is the family's shopping list. One powerful way of influencing what children eat is simply to make undesirable high-fat and high-sugar foods unavailable in the home. Taking this sort of action is not being restrictive but is setting boundaries (see Chapters 4 and 5 for a fuller exploration of the difference). It also avoids battles and conflict – if children grow up in an environment where only healthy foods are available they naturally expect to eat these at mealtimes and when they are hungry for snacks.

A family's access to healthy foods may not always be in their own hands. Families living in poverty are particularly disadvantaged – without a car it is difficult to go to a supermarket and stock up on healthy foods, some of which may also be more expensive than less healthy alternatives. Local shops often do not, or cannot, offer a plentiful supply of fruit and vegetables, as their shelf life is short. If these are offered, the quality is often poor and they are even more expensive than in the supermarkets.

Children's access to healthy foods can be further limited by their parents' inability to cook. Once part of most girls' education at school, nowadays many young parents – men and women – may not have been taught cooking skills or even experienced home cooking. The pressures of work, time and looking after young children can make it especially difficult to change a family's way of life.

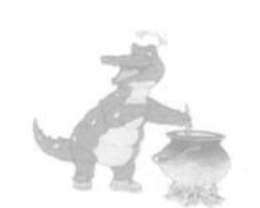

Within the home families differ in how much independent access to food children are allowed. In the past children would rarely go and help themselves to food from a cupboard or refrigerator, while now even very young children help themselves to food without asking. Clearly their choice is influenced by what sort of foods are available to them. At a more practical level, food also needs to be made accessible to young children by, for example, cutting up fruit and vegetables as easy to eat finger foods rather than presenting a whole item.

Key ideas

- Parents' knowledge, beliefs and food preferences influence their children's likes and dislikes as well as their eating habits
- Children are encouraged to eat and enjoy a varied diet when they see adults doing so
- Restricting certain foods has an unhelpful effect on children's preferences
- Babies' acceptance of weaning foods is influenced by flavours they meet during pregnancy and in breast milk
- Our food preferences are shaped by what we eat in the early years
- A healthy diet begins with the family's shopping list
- Even young children now have independent access to food so it is particularly important that their home offers a healthy eating environment
- Families living in poverty are particularly disadvantaged in their access to healthy foods

Encouraging healthy eating

Changing what we eat is arguably even more challenging than changing how we eat. It is therefore especially important that children are provided with healthy foods from the start. To do so requires knowledge about infant feeding, weaning, development of food preferences and changing requirements as children grow through the toddler and preschool years.

Breast or bottle?

The World Health Organisation clearly affirms that 'exclusive breastfeeding is nutritionally adequate for the first 6 months of an infant's life'. As a result, the Department of Health revised its guidance in 2004, recommending that:

- breastfeeding is the best form of nutrition for infants
- exclusive breastfeeding is continued for the first 6 months (26 weeks)
- solid foods are introduced at 6 months whether the infant is breast-fed, bottle-fed or a mixture of the two
- breastfeeding or formula feeding should continue beyond the first 6 months, with weaning foods appropriate in type and amount

Breastfeeding needs to be encouraged, at the same time as respecting parents' own choices. Knowing the health benefits may have some influence on the decision: gastrointestinal, respiratory and urinary tract infections are less likely and there is a reduced risk of allergies, obesity and type 1 diabetes in breast-fed babies. The added advantage of babies experiencing a variety of flavours through breastfeeding may encourage young mothers to eat a broad variety of healthy foods during breastfeeding (as well as pregnancy) in the knowledge that their baby is more likely to accept these foods at weaning.

There is often concern among both parents and professionals that breast milk is inadequate for some babies, and parents may need some reassurance that exclusively breastfeeding for six months poses no risk to their infant's health, growth and development. In fact, in this current epidemic of obesity we might well consider whether we should replace our anxieties about the inadequacy of breast milk with anxiety about the harm we may be doing by stopping breastfeeding prematurely and introducing formula before the age of 6 months.

In working with parents around early infant feeding, attention also needs to be paid to *how* the baby is fed, particularly if they are bottle-fed. Ideally, infants come to settle down to feeds every 3 to 4 hours, with reduced feeds in the night. When babies cry or regularly wake through the night and are fed, there is a danger that their milk intake leads to excessive weight gain. Indeed, this is one of the reasons why babies who wake often at night are more likely to develop obesity. Another issue may be babies' innate preference for sweet tastes such as milk – they often initially reject attempts to introduce water, leading their parents to believe that they do not like it. Parents may need to be reassured that offering water repeatedly will eventually lead to acceptance of it.

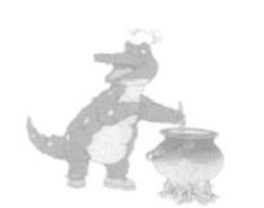

It is all too easy to over-feed babies who are bottle-fed, as it is tempting to encourage them to finish the bottle when they have stopped feeding. Breast-fed babies will stop when they have had enough, and are likely to be allowed to do so. It is helpful for parents who are bottle feeding to mimic breast feeding by looking for the baby's cues that they have had enough. This is an important part of responsive feeding (see Chapter 5). Encouraging parents not to overfill the bottle, to put it aside without taking into account how much has been taken, and certainly not encouraging the bottle to be emptied, avoids overriding the baby's cues and the unnecessary weight gain that can result.

The weaning process

Weaning can be an exciting milestone for parents or a time of anxiety and confusion. Community and health practitioners are often seen as an important source for guidance, so they are ideally placed to offer well-informed and timely support.

The choice of foods given at weaning is often unhealthy, being excessively high in fat and sugar with inadequate amounts of fruit and vegetables. The transition to family foods can worsen the situation. Surveys in the UK show that many infants rarely eat fruit and vegetables, and foods high in fat and sugar make a significant contribution to their diet.

Surveys of mothers indicate that they would like to receive both more information and more consistent information, and that confidence about weaning is often misplaced. While the majority of mothers believe their baby is eating a balanced diet, for example, many are not aware of the food groups, have limited knowledge of the variety of foods within the food groups, or believe they are providing sufficient iron but are unable to identify more than one good source of absorbable iron.

Parents have expressed a need for the following advice and support about weaning:

- the age at which to introduce particular foods
- what types of food to give
- how much food to give
- ideas for meal plans

In highlighting these needs they have identified the key dietary considerations so important in establishing good eating habits and avoiding the risk of obesity. Parents often have greater awareness of the issues than we give them credit for!

When to begin weaning
The recommendations are clear that weaning should start at 6 months of age. Waiting until then means that babies are likely to have a less energy-dense diet in the first

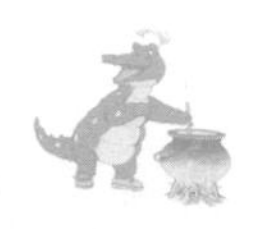

months of life, and there is good evidence that this practice is beneficial in reducing obesity: rates of obesity are known to be higher in children weaned before they are 16 weeks old.

The practice of early weaning has been a constant issue even when the recommended time to begin was between 4 and 6 months, so many parents may find it hard to accept and implement the new recommendations. Too often the following signs are often taken as signals that a baby is ready for weaning:

- waking at night after a period of sleeping through
- being unsatisfied after a full milk feed
- demanding more frequent milk feeds
- attempting to put objects in the mouth
- weight gain slowing or levelling out without a period of illness to explain why

In fact, caution is needed before assuming that the first four, at least, are indicators of readiness for solids. Advice is too often given by professionals, family or friends that the baby should be weaned – the best advice is to wait until the 6-month cutoff.

Introducing a healthy balanced diet

Exploring the extent of a parent's knowledge and skills in advance of weaning is a useful starting point. Introducing the 5 food groups is a simple and effective way of promoting healthy eating for babies and their families. The Eatwell plate developed by the Food Standards Agency has been adopted by HENRY as it promotes the idea of variety, balance and moderation. A healthy diet includes foods from all five groups, suggesting that there are no 'good' or 'bad' foods; it is the proportion of what we eat that is more or less healthy.

This way of working out what to eat is new to many people. It is clear, simple to use, and forms the basis for healthy eating. It may need to be explored in some detail in families unfamiliar with it. By recognising that a good weaning diet is important in laying down the foundations of healthy nutrition throughout life, parents may not only get their babies off to a good start but also be encouraged to eat more healthily themselves as they plan what to give the family to eat.

The first stages

Weaning introduces a baby to new tastes and textures and need contribute little at first to their nutrition, as milk continues to be the most important nutrient through most of the first year of life. At first the baby is likely to eat little, and may even appear confused or distressed by the novelty. This may be particularly true of bottle-fed babies, who will

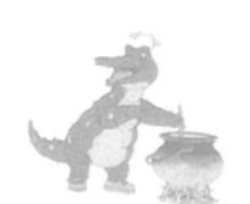

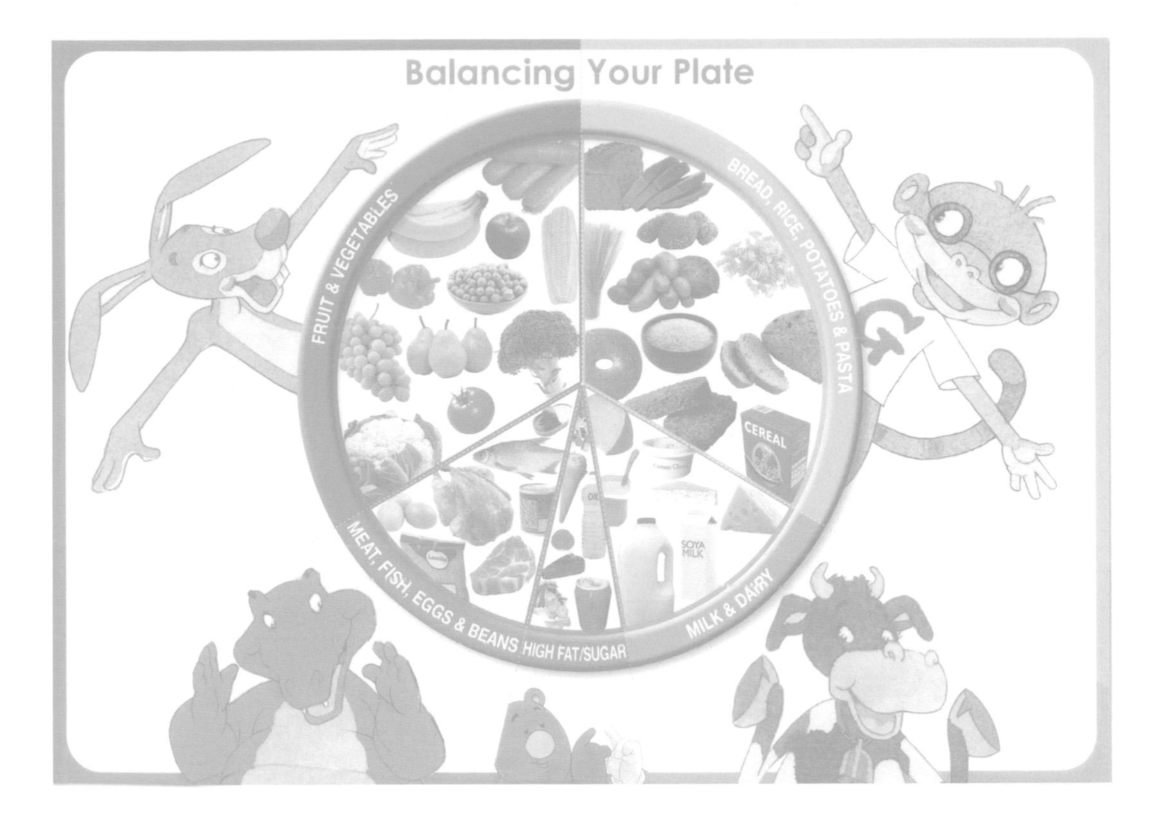

have experienced only one taste for the first few months of their lives. By contrast, the flavour of breast milk varies according to the mother's diet. Parents may need to be reassured that for a baby to react with surprise and even distaste is quite normal, and encouraged to approach feeding with a light touch (see below).

Babies gradually come to rely on solids to meet their nutritional needs, and make up the shortfall provided by their milk feeds. By the time they are fully weaned, they should be eating a wide variety of foods and participating in family meals and snack-times.

Nutritional recommendations

There are some specific nutritional recommendations of relevance to babies and toddlers. Breast or formula milk remains an important part of their diet, and needs to be continued to the age of 12 months, though 'door-step' milk may be used in cooking from the age of 6 months. As babies have small stomachs and need energy for growth, full-fat milk is then recommended until they are 2 years old. Full-fat dairy products such as yoghurt, non-sweetened fromage frais and cheese are also a helpful source of energy. Beyond the age of 12 months children need no more than 1 pint (approximately 500 ml) of milk a day: babies who are heavy milk drinkers often go on to become overweight. From the age of two years semi-skimmed milk – which has a lower fat content but similar vitamin A and D content – can be introduced.

FOODS TO TRY

First foods to try
- fortified baby cereals (providing iron and zinc)
- mashed cooked vegetable – carrot, parsnip, sweet potato
- mashed banana, avocado, cooked apple or pear
- baby rice mixed with the baby's usual milk

Second-stage foods
- mashed meat, fish, chicken
- mashed lentils, split pulses
- full-fat dairy products – yoghurt, fromage frais, custard

It is best to avoid fruit juices or baby drinks. They allow babies to become accustomed to sweet drinks, are not good for their teeth, and animal research tells us that they produce metabolic changes that promote the laying down of fat. If babies learn to drink water they are likely to be content to drink it when they are older, so it is best to offer only water or breast or formula milk between meals. Babies can learn to drink from a feeding cup early on in weaning. As drinking from a bottle encourages excessive drinking and dental caries, it is advisable to discontinue bottles as soon as the baby can manage a feeding cup comfortably.

If juice is given it should be well diluted (1 part fruit juice to 4–5 parts water). Soft drinks such as fruit squashes and carbonated drinks should not be offered. They increase the energy content of the diet without contributing any nutritional benefit. As with other sweet foods, their sugar and acidity promote dental caries. Drinks containing artificial sweeteners (diet drinks) are also not recommended.

Sugars are, however, an important source of energy at this stage, and are contained naturally in milk, fruits and vegetables. Adding sugar is not recommended as it leads to an excessively sweet tooth and dental caries later in life. Foods rich in sugar such as confectionery, cakes and chocolate are also best avoided. Parents who themselves have a sweet tooth may find it hard to accept that the natural sweetness in food will satisfy their baby, but may well recognise that it is better for their babies not to be encouraged to develop a taste for sweetness. Fried foods and those high in fat such as crisps and processed meat products are also best avoided.

Finger foods

By the age of 7 months a baby can usually manage finger foods such as small pieces of fruit, vegetables or toast. These introduce new tastes and textures and have the extra

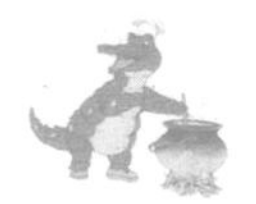

advantage that the baby learns to feed himself – an important stage in developing independence.

Parents can encourage their baby to chew, even if teeth have not yet come through, by offering raw or cooked green beans, carrot sticks, cubes of cheese, toast, breads including pitta bread, slices of banana and peeled apple. Some babies prefer from the outset food with 'handles' that they can hold to mashed foods offered on a spoon.

Using family food

Exploring how to give a baby the food that is being prepared for the rest of the family has two benefits: it offers an opportunity to reflect on how healthily the family as a whole is eating, and encourages the idea that introducing solids to the baby need not involve a lot of extra work. Family foods may need to be adapted for the baby as they need to be soft enough to be mashed, and cooked without the addition of salt or sugar.

Parents' suggestions for introducing suitable foods can be discussed in the light of healthy eating guidelines. An added bonus of this approach is establishing the principle that children eat ordinary food – that there is no need for one range of foods for children and another for adults (whatever the food industry would like us to believe).

Increasing acceptance of new foods

Research indicates that the wider the variety of foods the baby is exposed to in the early weeks and months of weaning, the greater the chances that these foods will be accepted, contributing to the overall quality of the diet throughout childhood. Gradually increasing the repertoire of foods offered leads to the baby eating a wide range of foods from each of the 4 main food groups. We need not regard rejection of a particular food as a sign of dislike. A baby's initial reaction is often to reject food as a result of the physiological thrusting action of the tongue or if the food offered is not sweet – a taste for which infants have an innate preference. It may take ten or more attempts on separate occasions before a baby will accept an unfamiliar food.

While it is helpful to encourage babies to accept new foods by repeatedly offering them, it is also important not to insist that a baby eats a particular food – time will tell us whether or not familiarity leads to acceptance or a baby genuinely does not like a particular taste (see discussion of feeding styles in Chapter 5).

How much, how often

At first, solids should be offered once a day, increasing to twice and then three times a day. It is best to introduce only one new food at a time so that any food intolerances can be identified more easily. As the baby eats more solid foods, the milk intake will start to

reduce. Babies will want to breastfeed less often, and the number of bottles for those on formula feed should be reduced, though formula milk should still be given until the end of the first year.

Many parents are anxious about how much they should expect the baby to eat, and are glad of reassurance that the body knows best – all we have to do is be sensitive to the cues they give about when they are hungry, need a pause or are full (see Chapter 5). Babies should not be expected to eat a prescribed amount – or even the same amount each day.

Portion sizes

There is good evidence that the rise in levels of obesity in Western countries is a result not only of a change in the types of food that we eat but also because portion sizes have increased. There is a common misconception about how much children need to eat. This is clear from some of the mealtime observations we have made; parents themselves comment on this when they view a recording of their own child's meal. Those who are unfamiliar with sensible portion sizes may worry unnecessarily that their young child is not eating enough, and try any tactic to encourage them to eat more.

Parents are often reassured to learn about suitable portion sizes, and to discover that the best guide to whether their baby or child is eating enough is to look at their growth pattern, development and energy levels over time rather than how much they eat in a day. The chart gives portion sizes that are reasonable to offer young children to satisfy their requirements and avoid excessive weight. Many people are surprised at the size of the portions. It is important to remember that they are only a guide – children's own hunger and fullness cues should determine whether they need more.

It is helpful to use smaller plates and bowls for young children's meals than those used for adults; they are a reminder that children need smaller portions.

As the baby gets older

When the baby is eating a sufficient quantity, foods from different food groups can be offered in the same meal. By now the baby should be learning to fit in with the family by eating three minced or chopped meals a day as well as milk. The baby can be included in the family mealtime routine, being fed while other members of the family are also eating.

In addition the baby should have a healthy sit-down snack between meals. These should not be given to replace a meal the child has declined to eat, but should be thought of as mini-mealtimes in their own right. Nutritious snacks also come from the 4 main food groups (fruit, vegetables and bread make good snacks) rather than from the high fat/high

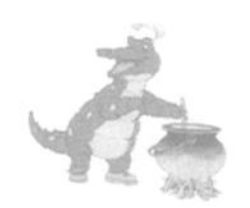

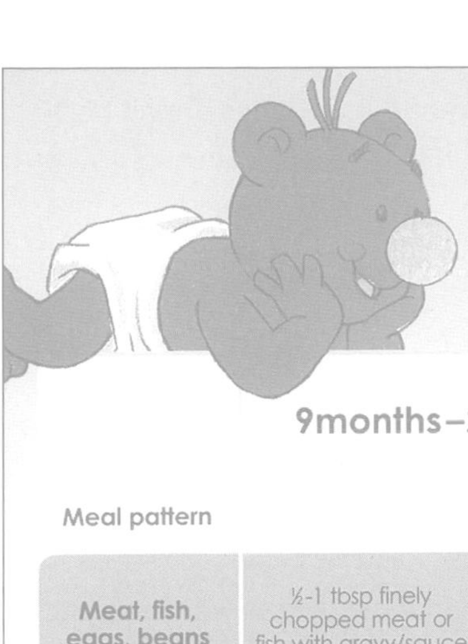

How big is a portion?

The HENRY guide to portion sizes for the under 5s

	9months–2yrs	2yrs–3yrs	3yrs–5yrs
Meal pattern		3 small meals plus 2 snack times	
Meat, fish, eggs, beans and other non dairy protein	½-1 tbsp finely chopped meat or fish with gravy/sauce 1 egg 1 tbsp baked beans	1½ tbsp chopped meat or fish 1 fish finger 1 egg 1-2 tbsp baked beans 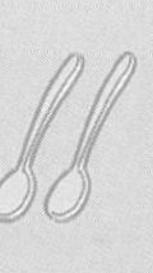	1 slice of meat 1 piece of fish 1 egg 1-2 fish fingers 2 tbsp baked beans 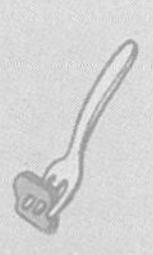
Fruit (1 portion is about a child's handful)	½ small apple or pear 1 small plum 1 small slice of melon 2-3 strawberries or grapes 	½ apple or pear 1 small plum 1 slice of melon 4-5 strawberries or grapes 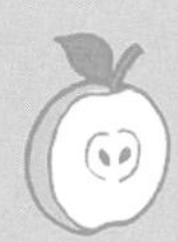	1 small apple or pear 1 plum 1 slice of melon 6 strawberries or grapes 
Vegetables	1 tbsp soft or mashed vegetables eg carrots, courgettes or broccoli 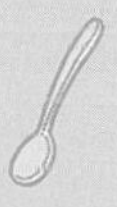	1-2 tbsp vegetables 1 small chopped salad 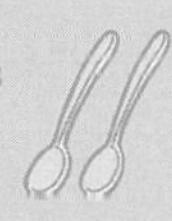	2-3 tbsp vegetables 1 small salad 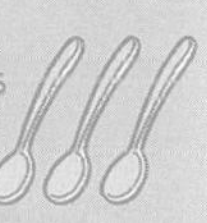
Bread, rice, potatoes, pasta and other starchy foods	½-1 slice bread 1 tbsp mashed potato or rice 3-4 chips 1 tbsp porridge or cereal 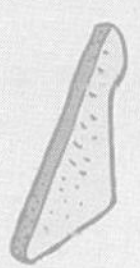	1 slice bread 1-2 tbsp mashed potato, rice or pasta 5-6 chips 1-2 tbsp porridge or cereal 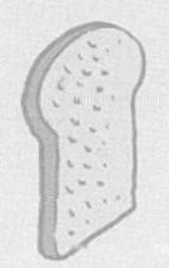	1-2 slices bread 2-3 tbsp mashed potato, rice or pasta 6-8 chips 2-3 tbsp porridge or cereal 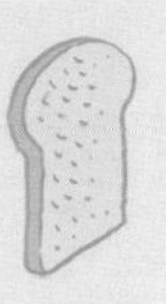
Milk and dairy foods – no more than 1 pint milk (600 mls) each day	3 dice-size pieces of cheese 2 tbsp yoghurt or custard 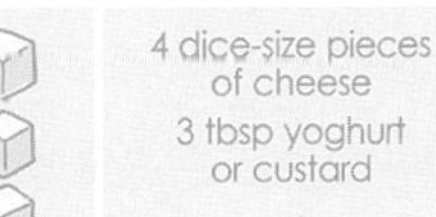 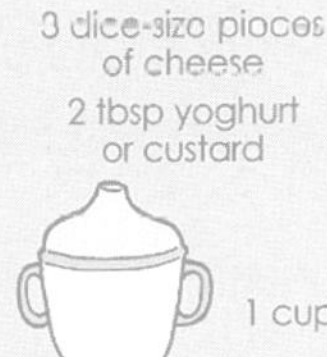 1 cup full fat milk	4 dice-size pieces of cheese 3 tbsp yoghurt or custard 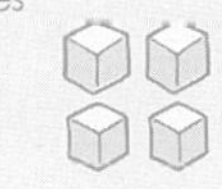 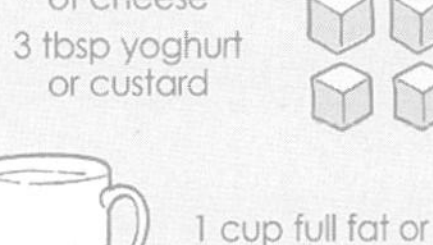 1 cup full fat or semi-skimmed milk	5 dice-size pieces of cheese 1 small carton yoghurt 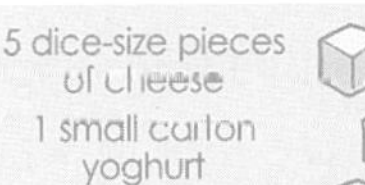 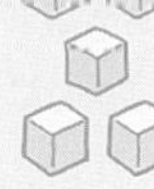 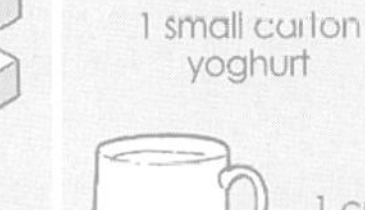 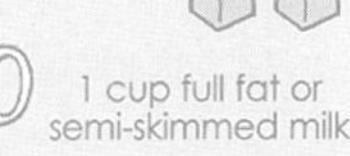 1 cup full fat or semi-skimmed milk
Foods and drinks high in fat and/or sugar	1 biscuit Small piece of cake 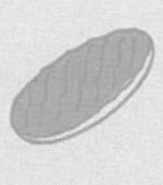	1 biscuit Small piece of cake 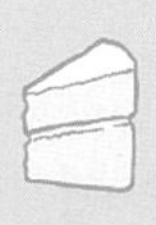	2 biscuits Medium piece of cake 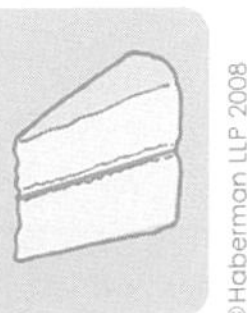

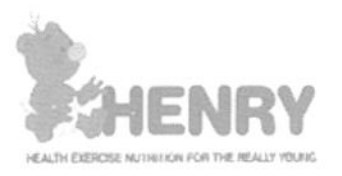

One item in each food group makes a portion; amounts are given in tablespoons (tbsp)
Adapted from Nutritional Guidance for Early Years. Scottish Government Publication

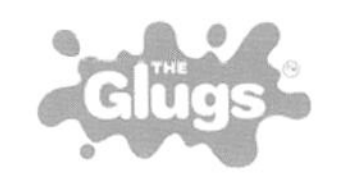

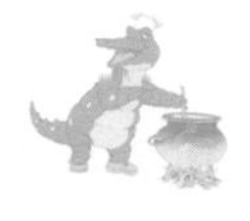

sugar group – crisps, cakes, biscuits, confectionery, ice cream and soft drinks are all best avoided. Giving these energy-dense snacks can make a significant contribution to young children putting on too much weight.

Toddlers

Some of the conflict around mealtimes that often arises with toddlers is due to a lack of understanding about how they eat. Babies grow very rapidly, particularly in the first six months; by toddlerhood their growth rate has slowed down, so they need to eat relatively less despite the fact that they are larger and more active. Toddlers also often eat sporadically, being hungry at one meal and wanting to eat less at the next. Looking at what a toddler eats over the course of a few days, rather than worrying about how much they eat at any one meal, usually reassures parents. It also helps them stay responsive to the toddler's own signals about hunger and fullness, which will enable them to relax and make them less likely to over-encourage or coerce their child into eating more than the child needs.

Preschool children

Preschool children should move to eating the family diet, though of course still with child-sized portions (see chart). Their eating patterns should now reflect those of the rest of the family, so they are familiar with a wide range of foods and able to eat independently by the time they start school.

Babies and children who are gaining too much weight

All the issues discussed in this chapter are of particular importance if the child is already showing unhealthy weight gain. This is discussed in more detail in Chapter 8. The goal is to reduce the rate of weight gain while maintaining growth in terms of height.

RECOMMENDATIONS FOR BABIES WHO ARE GAINING TOO MUCH WEIGHT

- Make sure that portion sizes are appropriate
- Offer food on smaller plates
- Reduce high-fat and high-sugar foods to a minimum
- Offer vegetables if hungry
- Try to cut out night-time feeds
- Consider replacing full-fat milk with skimmed milk beyond the age of 12 months*
- Allow no sweetened drinks
- Ensure that food is eaten only in the context of mealtimes, and that it is not given as treats or rewards

* Dietetic advice is needed in this circumstance as vitamin supplementation may be required

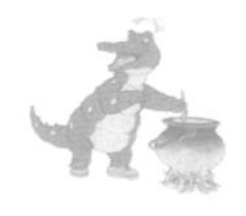

The starting point is to ensure that the baby has a healthy balanced diet and that their eating patterns follow the guidelines given in Chapter 5. For many babies this will be enough for their weight gain to return to the healthy range. The greater the rate of weight gain, the more important it is that the family adopts the recommendations shown below.

If weight gain continues at a very excessive rate (see Chapter 8), the advice of a dietitian is needed. Introducing any sort of weight-reducing diet requires specialist supervision, and a paediatric opinion is also needed to ensure that the child does not have a medical cause for their weight gain.

Key ideas

- Exclusive breast-feeding for at least 6 months is the healthiest choice
- When babies are bottle-fed it is helpful to feed responsively and mimic the way that breast feeds are given
- It is best to start weaning when the baby is 6 months old
- The 5 Eatwell food groups are a useful guide when planning meals for anyone in the family
- Snacks are best taken from the 4 main food groups and foods in the high-fat/high-sugar group avoided
- Foods and flavours experienced in the early years influence our likes and dislikes later in life
- Apart from milk, water is the best drink for babies and juice is unnecessary and undesirable
- Young children may need to be offered a new food up to 10 times before they accept it
- Portion sizes are often too large – it is better to use a small plate, give smaller portions and offer second helpings if the child is still hungry

Exploring the issues with parents

Exploring the diet of a young child and the family can be a delicate matter, particularly if the parents are sensitive about the problem of obesity for themselves or their children. A common perception is that health professionals tend to be judgemental so there is, as

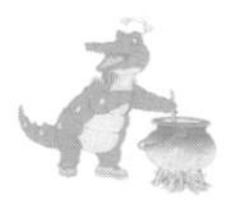

ever, a real need to take the time to earn parents' trust, to seek out their strengths and to build on these rather than making them feel defensive as a result of our actual or implied criticism.

Weaning is a significant milestone in a baby's life, and many parents are glad to receive support at this time. It therefore offers a golden opportunity to find out what parents already know about healthy eating and whether they are aware of the risks of obesity. Some parents will already be knowledgeable, and need only be reassured, while others may need more support through the weaning period.

We are almost all aware that we should eat 5 portions of fruit and vegetables each day. Despite this, in the UK we eat on average only about 2 portions per day. Clearly, many of us have knowledge that we do not apply! This should alert us to the fact that simply giving information to parents is unlikely to bring about change: we need to engage parents, harness their knowledge, and help them find their own motivation for ensuring that their families eat healthily.

The question is often more about how to introduce different types of foods into the family diet than lack of knowledge. Encourage the parent to lead the discussion about this so you can discover what they already know, and affirm their knowledge. Providing relevant extra tips as the parent identifies the need for them is more helpful than telling them at the outset what we believe they need to know. They are more likely to implement new ideas if these feel part of a process of exploration rather than their being bombarded with information.

We need to be extra sensitive in families where there is little sign of home cooking taking place; there is no point in offering advice on what to cook if a parent does not know how to cook. It may be helpful, when the parent indicates that they would be glad of this, to show them how to cook one or two basic meals, and even to provide cooking utensils. Children's Centres and other settings offer basic cooking courses for young parents, so it is worth finding out about these and perhaps, when the time is right, suggesting that a parent might like to join a class.

Food recall and food diaries

If there are concerns around food or weight gain, it can be helpful to explore with the parent quite precisely what their child eats and drinks over the course of a day.

Start by asking what the child has eaten on waking, and work steadily through the day, asking the parent whether they would like you to jot down notes so you can look at the whole picture together. It can help to prompt with questions such as 'What did the child

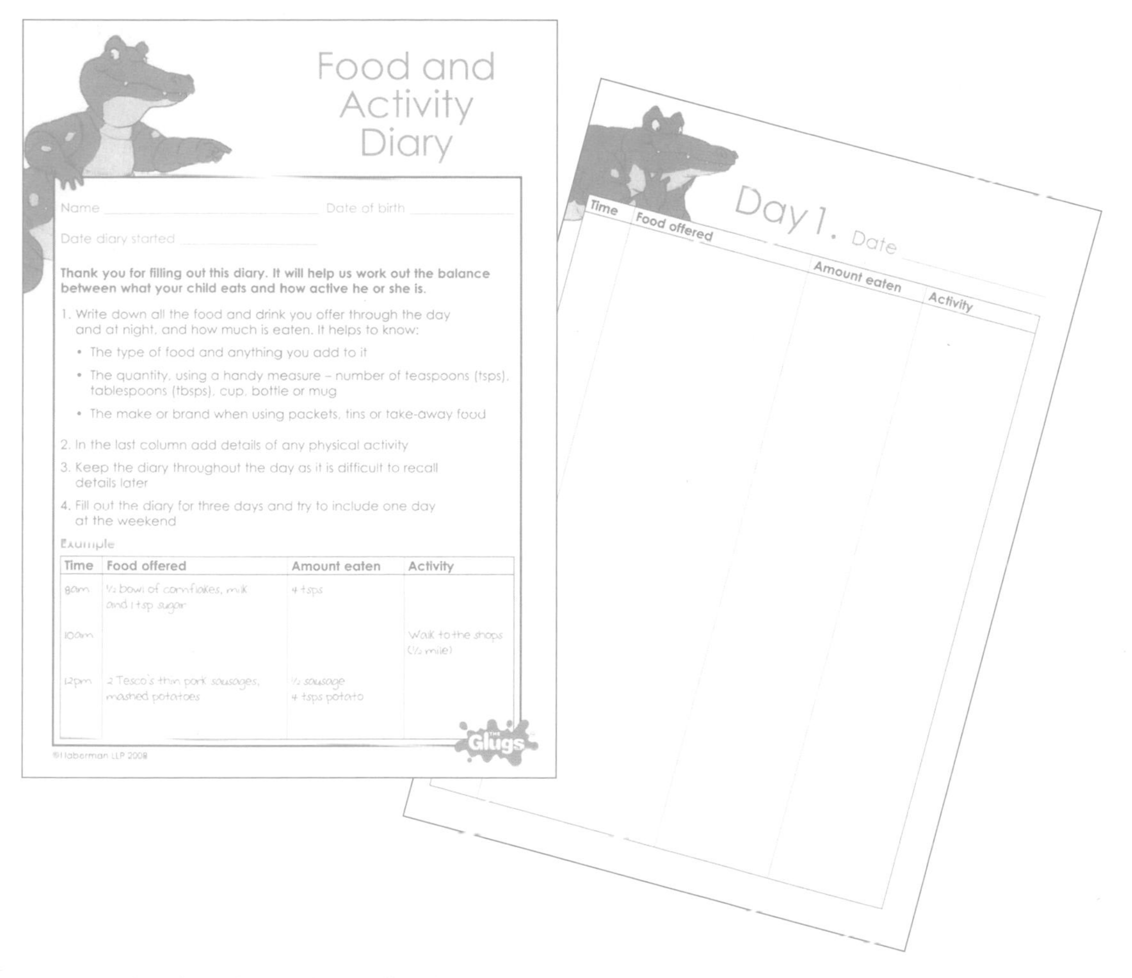

Food and Activity Diary

Name ______________________ Date of birth ____________

Date diary started ______________

Thank you for filling out this diary. It will help us work out the balance between what your child eats and how active he or she is.

1. Write down all the food and drink you offer through the day and at night, and how much is eaten. It helps to know:
   - The type of food and anything you add to it
   - The quantity, using a handy measure – number of teaspoons (tsps), tablespoons (tbsps), cup, bottle or mug
   - The make or brand when using packets, tins or take-away food
2. In the last column add details of any physical activity
3. Keep the diary throughout the day as it is difficult to recall details later
4. Fill out the diary for three days and try to include one day at the weekend

Example

Time	Food offered	Amount eaten	Activity
8am	½ bowl of cornflakes, milk and 1 tsp sugar	4 tsps	
10am			Walk to the shops (½ mile)
12pm	2 Tesco's thin pork sausages, mashed potatoes	½ sausage 4 tsps potato	

eat next?' rather than asking what he ate for any particular meal, to make sure that any snacks are included. The process should allow you to gain a picture of:

- the content and size of meals
- what has been offered and what has been eaten
- the timing and structure of mealtimes
- what snacks and drinks have been offered
- any issues or difficulties that have arisen

Parents may, as an alternative, find it helpful to keep a diary and record what their child has eaten. Three days is generally the length of time that yields useful information without becoming too tedious an exercise. An example of a food diary is shown in the figure. The diary sheet has not been divided into meals, but allows parents to record any food/drink taken. This helps to give a full picture of everything eaten rather than just food eaten at mealtimes. The column for activity helps to reinforce the importance of balancing intake and output.

You will need to explain carefully to the parent how to fill in the diary – for example, clarifying that they need to write down what the child has eaten as well as what has been offered. When the diary has been completed, you will usually find that you can interpret it yourself, but in situations where there is concern that there are inadequate nutrients (e.g. iron or calcium) being eaten, you may need the help of a dietitian.

Sharing feedback

The way of sharing feedback described in Chapter 5 is a helpful way to review the recall list or food diary, as well as a mealtime. This involves letting the parent take the lead by seeking their opinion before you offer yours. Looking at what the baby has eaten in relation to the 5 food groups can help to highlight what the parent is already doing to feed the child healthily, and what they might be able to do to improve the child's diet. Exploring in a straightforward way how our bodies use foods from the different groups is of interest to some parents, too.

Whether you and the parent decide to use recall or a diary, it is important also to focus on portion sizes when you review it together. You may wish to ask them to show you the size of the crockery and cutlery they are using, as this is a practical way to discuss appropriate portion sizes. The portion size chart may be helpful in your discussion.

Observation of a mealtime

In Chapter 5 we suggested that it might be helpful to observe a mealtime. While this is generally used to explore feeding styles and eating patterns, it is also a good opportunity to see what and how much the child is being offered to eat, and the nutritional quality of the meal. If relevant, this can also be explored with the parent in the feedback discussion.

Endword

Nature provides all the food we need to build, repair and fuel our bodies. In a world of confusing information, fluctuating food prices, aggressive marketing by the food industry, constant availability of unhealthy food products, shortage of time or skill, it can sometimes seem daunting to provide healthy food for the family. We have looked in this chapter at the principles of healthy eating for babies, young children and families. These are in fact relatively straightforward: providing young children with reasonable amounts of different types of healthy foods will stand them in good stead and ensure that they maintain a healthy weight as they grow. This is particularly true, both for children of all ages and for adults, if what we eat is balanced in another way – with how active we are. This is the subject of the next chapter.

References, further reading and resources

American Heart Association, Gidding SS, Dennison BA et al. Dietary Recommendations for Children and Adolescents: A Guide for Practitioners. *Pediatrics* 2006; 117: 544–559

Birch L & Dietz W (eds). *Eating Behaviours of the Young Child – prenatal and postnatal influences on healthy eating* American Academy of Pediatrics 2008

Crawley H. *Eating well for under-5s in child care: nutritional and practical guidelines / training materials* The Caroline Walker Trust 2006

Fisher JO and Birch LL. Feeding children in an environment of plenty: lessons from the laboratory in *Eating Behaviours of the Young Child – prenatal and postnatal influences on healthy eating* Eds Birch L & Dietz W. American Academy of Pediatrics 2008 pp 141–156

Fisher JO. Liu Y et al. Effects of portion size and energy density on young children's intake at a meal *American Journal of Clinical Nutrition*. 2007; 86:174–9

Mennella J.J., Jagnow, C.P. et al. Prenatal and postnatal flavor learning by human infants *Pediatrics* 2001; 107:E88

National Institute for Health and Clinical Excellence *Clinical Guideline* 43 Obesity Guidance 2006

Northstone K. Rogers I. Emmett P. ALSPAC Team Study. Avon Longitudinal Study of Pregnancy and Childhood. Drinks consumed by 18-month-old children: are current recommendations being followed? *European Journal of Clinical Nutrition* 2002; 56:236–44

World Health Organisation, UNICEF Global strategy for infant and young child feeding. WHO report 2003

Websites

The Caroline Walker Trust
http://www.cwt.org.uk

The Food Standards Agency
http://www.food.gov.uk

The Eatwell plate
http://www.food.gov.uk/healthiereating/eatwellplate

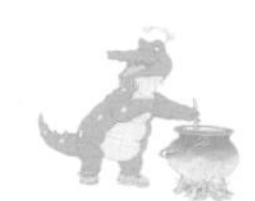

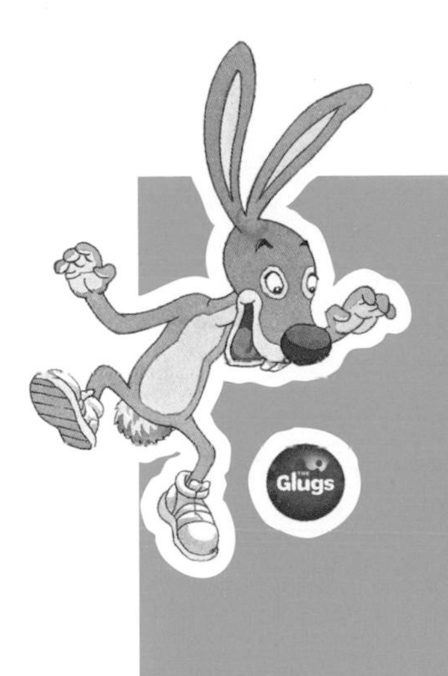

Being active

7

A healthy way of life is an active way of life. Being careful about what we eat and how we eat it is only half the equation – the energy we take in needs to be balanced by the energy we expend. For many families the challenge of making changes around family eating patterns is matched by that of developing an active family lifestyle. Many people do not regard being active as a priority, and unfortunately the less exercise we take, the less we feel like taking. The challenge is increased for those who are uncomfortably overweight or live in a flat or unsafe neighbourhood far from a park or other facilities. The limited amount of time available for busy working parents can also be a problem. Helping parents meet their children's need to be active from babyhood thus requires as much sensitivity and patience as the other key lifestyle areas.

In this chapter we will explore:

- the benefits of an active life
- the crucial part that parents play
- influences and constraints on opportunities for activity
- ways to meet children's need for activity – without spending large sums
- the question of TV
- how to encourage active families

Activity – the benefits and influences

Most of us live in an unnatural environment, where we do not need to grow our food, where machines do the physical work and vehicles carry us where we need to go. Toddlers are strapped into buggies and car seats, children in school are expected to sit still for long periods, and many of us go on to jobs that require us to do the same, whether at a supermarket checkout or a desk. It is then all too easy to spend much of our leisure time

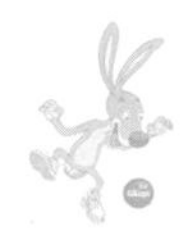

being passively entertained – perhaps sitting and watching other people taking part in sporting activities.

Until recently just the everyday activities needed to keep us alive would also have kept us relatively fit either out at work or running a home. Nowadays, building physical activity into the daily routine is something that is not always easy to do. Yet a reasonable level of fitness is essential for both our physical and our emotional health.

Why be active?

The benefits of exercise go beyond simply keeping weight in check. Physical activity increases adults' fitness, improves emotional health, lowers cholesterol levels and reduces the risks of heart disease and diabetes. This has been shown to be true for overweight and obese individuals even if they do not actually lose weight.

There are benefits during childhood too, and some parents may not be familiar with these. It is worth encouraging them to think about the fact that, for example, their children may sleep more soundly and be happier and easier to manage if they are active during the day.

BENEFITS OF AN ACTIVE LIFE

- stronger bones
- stronger muscles
- heart and lungs work well
- reduced risk of cardiovascular disease
- easier weight maintenance/reduction
- more energy
- mental alertness
- emotional well-being
- improved sleep

Parents and carers

Children are naturally active, and need plenty of opportunities to develop physically, gain skills and explore imaginative play. They usually delight in physical activity, particularly in the context of the family. This pleasure can be affected by a number of influences that can also determine how active children are as they grow older and on into adult life.

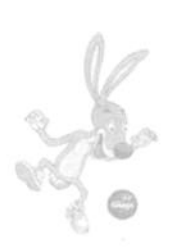

Arguably the strongest influence are parents and carers who shape their children's activity levels and also their enjoyment, attitudes and willingness to be active. They do this through modelling active and sedentary behaviour, their parenting style in relation to activity and their expectations.

Parents who enjoy being active naturally pass on the pleasure to their young children. Just as in the development of eating patterns and enjoyment of food, they offer a model for how to spend leisure time, how to relax and how to be active. The way they play with their children, and their attitude towards games and other forms of exercise, influences not only how active the children are, but also their ability to take turns and ultimately to participate in team sports. When adults dislike or are unaccustomed to being active, the message is likely to conveyed that physical activity is unimportant or a chore rather than a pleasure.

In Chapter 4 we considered the different styles of parenting according to how much parents are in charge within the family and how responsive they are to their child's wants and needs. The four styles – authoritative, authoritarian, indulgent and neglectful – have an impact in the area of physical activity too. Parents who adopt an indulgent or neglectful approach tend to have difficulties in setting fair limits, and may well permit or condone excessive screen-time at the expense of activity. Parents who tend towards an authoritarian approach may well ensure that their children are active. However, if they overly direct and control play, insist on the child taking part in activities they do not enjoy, or are over-focused on achievement and critical of the child's efforts, there is a danger that children may lose their enjoyment of physical activity. The authoritative approach, as in any aspect of parenting, is the optimal style. Parents who succeed in being responsive to their children and yet are capable of setting limits are most likely to help the children grow up to enjoy healthy exercise and balance it with an appropriate amount of food at mealtimes.

In order for parents to encourage their children to be active they also need to have a good understanding of their child's abilities, temperament and developmental stage. If parents try to encourage their child to run, jump, catch or kick a ball before they are mature enough to do so, everyone will become frustrated. This is also true if a child is clumsy, poorly coordinated or simply not temperamentally suited to boisterous play. Unless parents have realistic expectations their child is likely to feel a failure and will be in danger of losing both their enjoyment of activity and their self-esteem.

For some parents, there are real barriers to involving themselves in active play with their children. A parent with mental health issues may not be able to do this; nor may a parent whose own parents did not model an active and playful parent–child relationship. There may be other social and cultural pressures that get in the way.

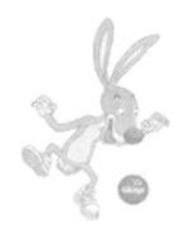

Influences and constraints

Even the most active families face constraints when it comes to giving children opportunities to spend a lot of time being active. Our environment has changed over the years, and where children in the past naturally engaged in activity through much of the day, they now spend much of the time being sedentary. They are less likely to be left to play on their own, even on home territory, let alone out of doors. The pressures of modern living also mean that they are likely to spend a good deal of time 'strapped in' and constrained when parents are going about daily activities such as shopping or travelling. Some babies and young children spend much of the day in pushchairs, baby bouncers, baby walkers and car seats. This not only limits their opportunities to be active but also leads to frustration, boredom and potential delays in their development; it is likely to encourage grazing, too.

The seductive screen

A special word needs to be said about television, which can be both a boon and a curse. It has been referred to as the flickering parent, as it is often used by busy parents to occupy and entertain their children. Unfortunately there is a correlation between obesity in children and the number of hours of television they watch. Watching more than 8 hours a week is linked to obesity, and recent studies in the UK show that young children on average watch as much as 3 hours television a day.

A number of explanations have been put forward as to why television has such a negative effect on the balance of children's lives. Watching TV is an exceptionally passive activity, and there is some evidence that children's metabolic rates are so reduced that they are as low as when they are asleep. If we add into the equation that children often snack on high-calorie food while they are watching, the balance, not surprisingly, is in favour of weight gain.

Key ideas

- Physical activity benefits health all through life
- Parents influence their children's enjoyment of activity through being active themselves
- Parenting styles have an important effect on children's attitudes towards active play
- Parents' mental health and circumstances affect children's opportunities to be active
- Modern living inhibits children's natural inclination to be active
- Television has a particularly powerful negative effect on children's lifestyles

7

Encouraging activity

As in other aspects of working with parents around issues of healthy living, we need to take a holistic approach and develop an awareness of the influences that affect a family's approach and attitudes. Leaping in with practical suggestions is unlikely to be helpful if inadequate attention is paid to the broader issues. Here we consider some of the questions parents may have, and information that may be helpful when encouraging parents and carers to adopt a more active way of life.

When can we begin to encourage activity?

Patterns of activity, just like eating patterns, have their roots in our earliest experiences. Parents do not always appreciate this. They may not have considered the fact that babies start to move long before they are born, and that once freed from the restrictions of the womb they need to begin to build the strength that enables them to develop in just one year from relatively inert newborns to the energetic powerhouse that is a toddler. Some parents instinctively encourage this natural urge to be active in the way they play with their babies; others do not. Engaging parents' interest in the way their baby develops, and how they can best help him/her grow into a strong and healthy child, can make a considerable difference.

Parents are likely to appreciate straightforward, relevant information about how babies develop. We can, for example, explain that strength builds from the head downwards. To

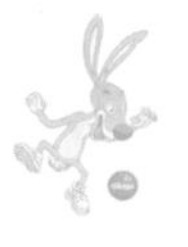

begin with, neck muscles strengthen so the head is held up and can turn – wanting to look around and see what is going encourages this. Next comes a strengthening of the trunk muscles so that eventually the baby can sit up, which greatly increases opportunities for play. Learning to crawl and walk follows on, often encouraged by frustration when objects the baby wants are out of reach. Helping parents to understand their baby's developmental progression will help them to recognise what activities are appropriate for the different stages the baby goes through.

Singing and baby dance are a particularly pleasurable way of promoting closeness and encouraging movement. Songs, rhymes and all kinds of music benefit babies from the very beginning (and even before they are born). As well as being enjoyable in their own right, they help a child's language development; children who know plenty of songs and rhymes when they start school are more likely to take readily to reading and writing. Most of us move naturally to the rhythm of rhymes and songs, and babies often love to be rocked, bounced and handled in a rhythmic way. With repetition, and as their muscles develop, they take an increasingly active part in the movements and sounds.

A safe exploring environment

Like chickens, young children thrive when they are free-range! We need to help parents recognise this. Baby carriers, prams, buggies and baby chairs all have their place, particularly if they are used in a way that encourages conversation and companionship. But if parents understand why even a young baby also needs time and space to move – to lie on a rug, unencumbered by clothes, both on his back and on his tummy, so that the neck and chest muscles can grow stronger – they are more likely to provide these opportunities. And as babies become more active, it is increasingly important to 'baby-proof' their surroundings so can explore safely.

Helping parents recognise that they will be meeting the child's need to explore, to move, to develop physically, will not only benefit the toddler's development but will also reduce the potential for conflict. A young child's natural curiosity far outstrips their capacity to navigate their surroundings or keep out of danger: exploring is the child's job, keeping them safe is the parent's job.

Some reminders for parents on how to create a safe home environment are given below.

While safety is a priority, it is also good to define space for an older child and have some props to promote play. This might include defining a stage in the living room for dance, or a pitch in the garden for games. The chart at the end of the chapter provides some examples of games that may be enhanced by defining space – either indoors or out.

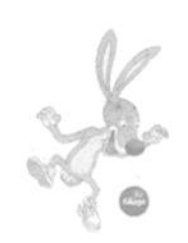

CREATING A SAFE ENVIRONMENT

- keep dangerous substances and precious objects out of reach
- pad sharp table corners
- supervise a baby learning to roll over, and when they are mobile enough to scoot and crawl
- have plenty of different objects to handle, chew and play with
- use a playpen for adults engaged on delicate tasks, or older children who want to play undisturbed, leaving the toddler to roam free
- find out what facilities for young children are available locally: Sure Start Children's Centres, for example, are friendly and well equipped

Toys and time to play

It is helpful to explore with parents ways of stimulating and appealing to all five senses – sight, hearing, smell, taste and touch. The toy industry is big business, and anxious parents provide a lucrative market. While toys can be exciting for young children, we can build parents' confidence by encouraging them to recognise how many everyday household objects will intrigue and entertain just as well and at a fraction of the cost.

If the question of cost comes up, you could help parents to think creatively by suggesting some examples of simple home made items. A mobile made by tying feathers, shiny paper stars or Christmas decorations onto a hanger to dangle above the changing mat will be just as interesting to a baby as a costly bought version, and the familiar alternative of wooden spoons and saucepans or tins may not be familiar to everyone. With a couple of ideas as examples, and a supportive conversation to build their confidence, many parents will find creative solutions to provide their children with alternatives to expensive toys. Steering them towards magazines, books or websites, toy libraries and other local activities, will also help them to take advantage of what is on offer.

What children need most of all is our loving attention and companionship. Part of the art of parenting is the balancing act between giving children our full attention, and doing household chores. For parents who work outside the home, this can be even harder to manage.

Once again, parents who enjoy being with their baby and enjoy playing are likely to devote time to it, while others may feel guilty and fear that they are wasting time if they spend it entertaining their baby or young child when chores are piling up. We can encourage parents to recognise that it is often possible to combine household tasks and play. We can blow bubbles and sing to a baby while we do the washing up. Young children love to copy what we do, and we can teach them useful skills while they help us to sweep

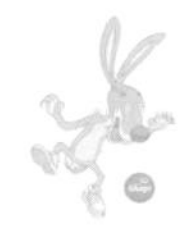

the floor, sort the washing, put away cutlery, and so on. A duster dance makes light of housework. There is always a payoff for making everyday chores fun, as a busy child is likely to be happier and more co-operative than a bored child. The chart at the end of the chapter gives suggestions of activities that parents may appreciate, and that require little in the way of equipment.

Relating as a family and child-led play

We need to be careful not to give the impression that parents should be directing their children's play all the time. Some time also needs to be devoted to child-led play, and sometimes a baby or young child will be happy just watching the world go by or playing on their own. Parents' attitudes to play may reflect their preferred feeding style, and your guidance can be similarly tailored both to build the parent's confidence in what they are already doing and to encourage them in playing with their child more enjoyably and perhaps more actively. Young children give us immediate and clear feedback on whether or not what we are doing meets their needs; learning to pick up the cues they send will increase parents' sensitivity to the way their children communicate, even as babies.

Physical activity can be a great opportunity for building family relationships. For some fathers in particular, it can provide a good way of feeling involved with their children. But it does require quality attention – flicking a ball towards a child while watching television is not likely to be engaging. Just as healthy eating patterns are promoted by eating together, so families need to play together.

Physical activity also provides an opportunity to encourage children's confidence and to praise and reassure them. This ensures that play with the family is a positive experience and is fun, and allows children to continue to try until they achieve. If expectations are inappropriate or children feel they have let their parents down, they may lose confidence and self-esteem. Ridiculing a child for poor co-ordination or being unable to play with a ball skilfully can easily have a negative impact in the longer term on their desire to take part in physical activity.

Parents may not appreciate that physical activity can help develop children's ability to communicate and relate as well as their coordination and capacity for imaginative play. Here are some examples of encouraging comments that promote positive interactions during play and can help the development of these skills, helping children to persevere when a task proves difficult.

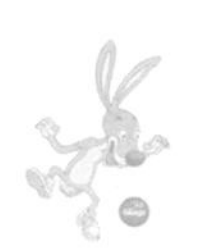

ENCOURAGING COMMENTS DURING PLAY

'It's fun playing with you'
'You're doing so well'
'Let's see if we can catch it'
'Let's roll it to each other'
'Fantastic! You caught it'
'Let's have another go'
'Nearly!'
'Great teamwork!'

Screen time

Television can have a huge impact on children's levels of activity, as well as affecting the development of their capacity for imaginative play. In recognition of this, the American Academy of Pediatrics has recommended that children under the age of 2 years should watch no television at all; older children should watch no more than 2 hours each day.

Left to their own devices, many children will opt for watching TV, particularly if the set is on all day, and it is up to parents to set limits for what programmes to watch and to provide alternative activities for children. There is a difference between a parent and young child actively watching a programme together, and then perhaps talking about it and doing an activity based on what they have seen, and the glazed passive watching that comes with hours of TV without any conversation or companionship. This of course applies to watching videos and DVDs as well.

Key ideas

- understanding babies' developmental progress helps ensure that expectations are realistic
- children don't need to be taught to be active and play – they just need a safe exploring environment
- everyday items and imagination do as well as expensive toys
- when physical activity is a positive experience, children develop both skills and confidence
- physical activity helps to build family relationships
- adults need to guide and limit children's TV viewing time
- children need exercise – any vigorous activity counts

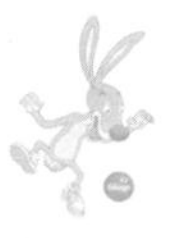

Exploring the issues with parents

A very young child is often the most active family member – indeed, many get into trouble for being lively when others want peace and quiet. In an active family the child's natural exuberance will be channelled constructively with outdoor play, rough and tumble games at home, and so on. But how often do we hear young children being criticised for running around in the supermarket? It is so easy to regard this sort of behaviour as naughtiness rather than recognising it as a healthy need to be active.

When working with young families we need to be aware of how physical activity is seen, and what may influence the children's attitudes and enjoyment. Providing ideas for games and play is likely to be more effective if we can take in the broader picture and be sensitive to parents' attitudes towards physical activity and the constraints they live under.

Encouraging parents to look at the activity levels of the family as a whole, and to consider whether a more active lifestyle would be in the family's interests, can lead to a shift in attitude and provide a catalyst for change. If the adults are sedentary, overweight or unaccustomed to being active, helping them to find their own motivation and to set realistic goals in the interests of the family's health may take time, but the health benefits – physical and emotional – can be considerable.

It is important to start by exploring parents' general attitudes to an active lifestyle for themselves and their families. If you have already discussed eating and mealtimes, you may have a sense of the style of parenting they favour. This may be a starting point for discussing physical activity, though some parents will have quite different attitudes to eating and play. Whatever their approach, the first task is to listen in order to identify and appreciate ways in which parents already enjoy interacting and playing with the baby/child. You will need to be sensitive to a parent's anxiety or reluctance to play, and it may be helpful to explore this too.

Observing how a parent responds to their baby/child (see Chapter 4) will give you clues about how comfortable they are together, and how playful their relationship is. Bear in mind that a parent may feel inhibited in your presence until a trusting relationship has been established, and may feel foolish behaving in a loving, intimate way with the baby. Modelling a playful approach yourself may help to put a parent at ease – though there is also the possibility of provoking a sense of inadequacy if the parent is less skilled at engaging with the baby than you are. It is important that you do not take over or let parents simply observe you, the expert, at play.

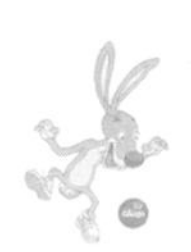

One needs to remember too that not all parents find it easy to play with their baby or young child. Exhaustion, depression, feeling overwhelmed, even not knowing what to do, may all play a part. Those whose parents did not play with them when they were young may have little sense of how to engage with young children and enjoy their company. For all these reasons we need to be sensitive in seeking parents' views and trying to gain a clearer idea of what issues they may have.

As ever, demonstrate respect towards parents by asking questions about what activities they and the baby/child do together, and which are most popular. Exploring together what is already happening, and showing appreciation for the parent's creativity, skills and expertise, will open up the discussion more quickly. Engaging a parent's curiosity about how babies and young children develop can lead to an invitation to provide factual information about developmental stages that can act as a springboard for further exploration of appropriate activities. It can also lead to a discussion about other activities that can be introduced to meet the baby's needs.

Television is an important issue to address, and can be a tricky subject to raise, as it is often adults' principal form of relaxation and entertainment as well as a way of keeping children occupied. A harassed or tired parent needs support, and acknowledgement of how challenging it can be to match young children's energy throughout the day. Discussing alternative activities for children and their parents in a way that genuinely explores and extends parents' point of view, engaging in a non-judgemental way rather than telling them what to do and leaving them feeling criticised or misunderstood, is a test of skill in applying the HENRY approach.

On a practical level, you could invite the parent to consider whether they might find it helpful to keep an activity diary (in the same way as food diaries can be helpful). This could be a trigger for discussion at another session, and perhaps the basis for setting goals and developing a strategy towards a more active family life. It is well worth developing your own folder of facilities and opportunities for young children in your local area so you can signpost parents towards them. The chart outlines some specific suggestions that parents might find helpful in thinking about how to provide more exercise for their children at home.

Endword

In looking at what constitutes a healthy lifestyle for young families, the E for Exercise in the HENRY approach is as important as the other elements. While many practitioners are concerned about nutrition, fewer take the other half of the energy balance into account to the same extent. Helping parents recognise the many benefits of an active lifestyle and the impact it has on children's behaviour and sleep patterns, and encouraging small steps

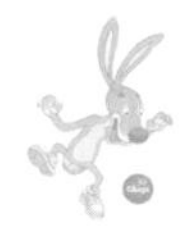

towards a more active lifestyle for the whole family, can improve family relationships as well as contributing to everyone's health. This topic lends itself to the HENRY approach; with support, parents will come to value their own ideas for ensuring that their children are active, and perhaps reach out to explore what is available for families in their own community such as the local Children's Centre.

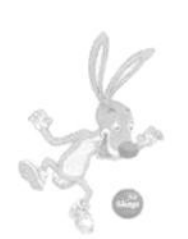

ACTIVE PLAY – IDEAS FOR PARENTS

BALL PLAY
You can use:
– A light ball
– A bean bag
– Rolled up socks can be soft and easier to catch!
– Plastic cones, cushions, tins or plastic beakers make good space markers

- Try playing catch together. To make it easier move nearer or to make it harder move further away
- Try throwing the objects into a box or laundry basket together. To make it easier move the box nearer or to make it harder move it further away
- Sit on the floor and roll the ball between you. Roll the ball between two space markers or cushions
- Use space markers as obstacles along a trail and try to kick the ball around the obstacles from start to finish

HIDE AND SEEK

- Hide balls or toys around the room and ask your child to find them and put them into a box or laundry basket
- To make it easier point to where they are or give clues
- To make it harder give your child a time limit by counting slowly. Next time they could try to beat their last time

BALLOONS
A balloon can be fun and moves more slowly than a ball (If you don't inflate it fully it's less likely to pop!)

- Try patting a balloon up in the air and keeping it up between you
- Make a 'net' with string and pat it back and forward over the top

RACES

- Make an obstacle course or race track with a start and finish line (you could use string or cushions) and play fun races
- Try different races hopping, skipping, on hands and feet, backwards, frog jumps or invent your own!

LET'S DANCE

- Put on some lively music – any music you like is fine
- Bounce your knees to the beat, twist your hips or make arm moves to the beat with your child
- Just let yourself go and don't worry about how it looks!

SCARF DANCING
You can use light floaty scarves or pieces of material like chiffon

- Show your child how to hold one in each hand and wave their arms to the music or make patterns in the air.
- Hold one end of the scarves each and have a dance together
- Play cheerleading – with scarves in each hand make strong punching arm movements to the sides and above your head. Add in some jumps and kicks if you like

SHOWTIME

- Play 'Dance Shows' by marking out a little stage with markers or cushions and let your child 'perform' a dance.
- They could choose their favourite music and dress up too if they like. Give them a round of applause when they finish.

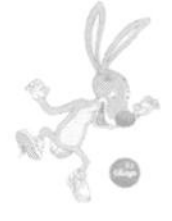

References, further reading and resources

Committee on Nutrition Policy Statement. Prevention of Pediatric Overweight and Obesity. *Pediatrics* 2003. 112 : 424–430

Committee on Public Education American Academy Of Pediatrics. Children, Adolescents, and Television *Pediatrics* 2001; 107: 423–426

Department of Health Physical activity, health improvement and prevention committee. *At least five a week: Evidence on the impact of physical activity and its relationship to health.* DH Report 2004

Featherstone S, Ingham K. *The Little Book of Outdoor Play: Little Books with Big Ideas* Featherstone Education 2001

Filer J. Healthy, *Active and Outside! Running and Outdoors Programme in the Early Years* David Fulton 2008

Gavin ML, Dowshen SA, Izenberg N. *Fit Kids: A practical guide to raising healthy and active children – from birth to teens* Dorling Kindersley 2004

Kaiser Family Foundation *The Media Family: Electronic media in the lives of infants, toddlers, preschoolers and their parents* Menlo Park, Calif. Kaiser Family Foundation 2006

Reilly JJ, Armstrong J et al for the ALSPAC Team. Early life risk factors for obesity in childhood: cohort study. *BMJ* 2005. 330: 1357–1359

Riddoch CJ, Mattocks C, et al. Objective measurement of levels and patterns of physical activity. *Archives of Disease in Childhood* 2007; 92: 963–9

Robinson TN Television viewing and childhood obesity *Pediatric Clinics of North America* 2001, 48, 1017–1025

Skinner, S. *Creative Activities for the Early Years* Paul Chapman Publishing 2007

Strong T, LeFevre D. *Parachute Games* Human Kinetics 1996

Vandewater EA. Linking TV viewing and children's obesity in *Eating Behaviours of the Young Child – prenatal and postnatal influences on healthy eating* Eds Birch L & Dietz W. American Academy of Pediatrics 2008 pp 101–122

Wilmes L, Wilmes D. *Parachute Play* Building Blocks 2000

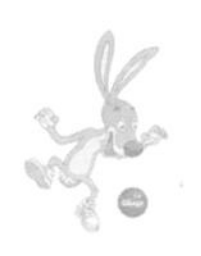

Websites

FUNdamental Movement Ideas
www.earlyyearsfundamentals.co.uk

Information, products and ideas for parents and teachers
http://www.earlychildhood.com

Start to Play – Youth Sport Trust resources
www.ystdirect.org.uk

Sure Start website – ideas for play and practical support
http://www.surestart.gov.uk/improvingquality/frameworks/birthtothreematters

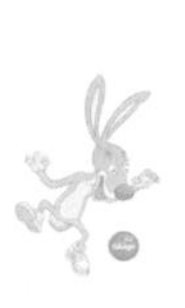

CLINICAL ISSUES

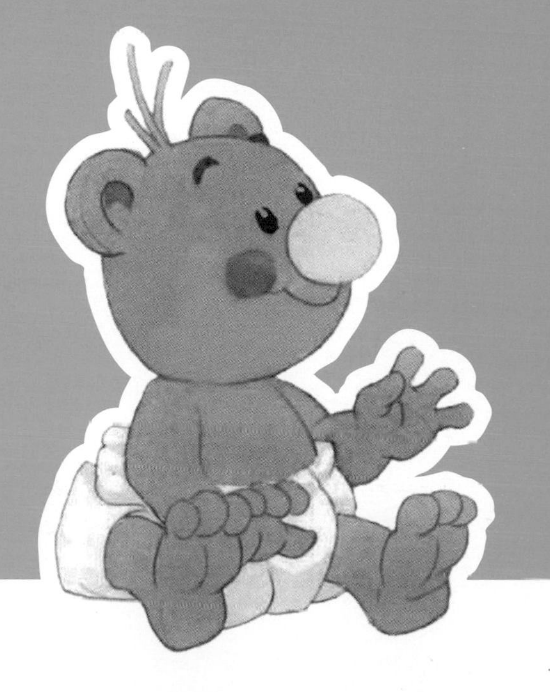

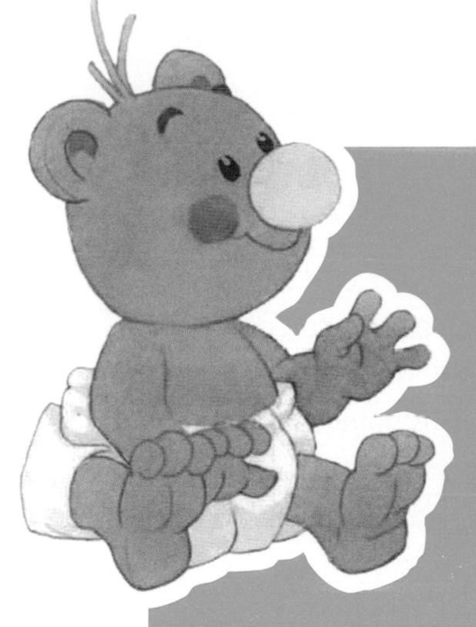

PART THREE

Obese babies and toddlers and other health concerns

This chapter is intended for health visitors and other practitioners who are likely to identify and work with families where babies and young children are already obese, are gaining weight rapidly or whose circumstances place them at particular risk of obesity. It is important that these children are identified early and provided with appropriate support, as it only gets harder to tackle obesity once it is entrenched. Examples of situations where children are at particular risk include developmental problems or disability, parents with mental health or learning difficulties, families living in poverty and those from certain ethnic backgrounds. At times you may also need to consider if there might be a medical cause for obesity or child protection concerns, and know when to involve other professionals.

The purpose of the chapter is to provide you with some direction to guide you in these more complex situations.

In this chapter we will explore:

- factors that increase a baby's risk of obesity later in life
- the clinical evaluation of a baby or child where obesity is an issue
- patterns of weight gain that suggest a baby is at particular risk
- how to work with babies and toddlers who are obese
- features that should alert you to the possibility of a medical cause for obesity
- the impact of developmental problems
- when obesity is a child protection issue
- parental issues, including parental mental health and parental obesity
- when to refer on

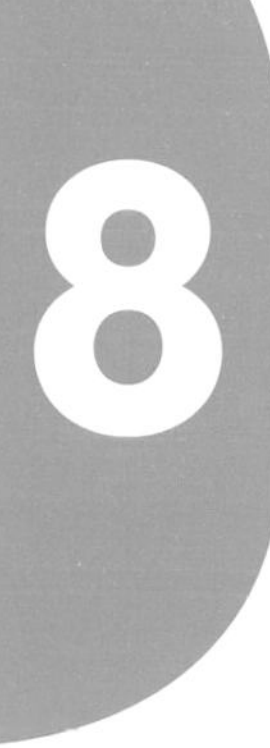

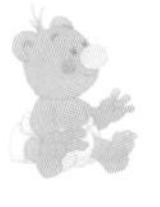

Your clinical assessment

Health professionals are generally comfortable and confident in identifying and working with parents around weight faltering and failure to thrive. They are often not so confident when it comes to working with obesity, although there are many similarities in approach. Just as when a baby shows poor weight gain, the baby who is large or is gaining weight excessively merits a clinical evaluation. This involves considering factors that increase a baby's risk of obesity, the possibility of a medical cause, the type of parenting approach the parents have adopted, and the child's home environment.

Factors that increase a baby's risk of obesity

The most important factors that influence the development of obesity are familial, though socioeconomic factors also play a part, as do a baby's weight and pattern of weight gain. Despite popular belief, genetic, metabolic or hormonal causes are very rare, though you do need to be alert to features that suggest there may be a problem. Conditions indicating that a baby may be at higher risk for obesity are shown in the box.

CONDITIONS THAT INCREASE THE RISK OF OBESITY

Common conditions

- Rapid weight gain in the first year
- Large babies (>98th centile for weight)
- Parental obesity (particularly if both are obese)
- A family history of obesity
- Obesity during pregnancy

Socioeconomic factors

- Bottle feeding
- Poverty
- Certain ethnic groups

Medical conditions

- Some syndromes, e.g. Down's syndrome
- Hypothalamic and genetic obesity syndromes, e.g. Prader Willi Syndrome
- Physical disability

There is no doubt that the strongest risk factor for obesity is parental obesity, and beyond that a wider family history. The risks are high – figures suggest that if one parent is obese the child has a 40% chance of being obese themselves, and if both parents are obese this

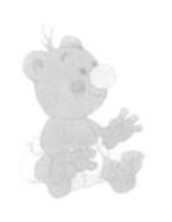

increases to 80%. The reasons for this are twofold. Parents give their children not only the genes that contribute to body size and shape, but also the home environment. We cannot do anything about babies' genetic heritage, so the focus of our work has to be on adjusting the home environment.

Children's risks increase further if there are other close family members who are obese or when there is a family history of early heart disease or diabetes in conjunction with obesity. Worryingly, it is now known that maternal obesity during pregnancy also has an independent long-lasting effect on babies' later weight gain. This gives a clear message that family planning advice should encourage mothers to achieve a healthy weight before they become pregnant. Weight loss is of course not advisable once the pregnancy is under way.

The family's social setting is also important. Ethnicity has an influence both in terms of a particular vulnerability to obesity and its complications, and the extent to which obesity is viewed as a problem that needs to be addressed. Poverty has a large impact too, placing disadvantaged children at particular risk, and far greater challenges for families seeking opportunities for activity and healthy food options.

Exploration and observations

In Chapter 3 we looked at issues that are relevant to explore when you and parents are thinking about healthier lifestyle options. These are particularly relevant when a baby or young child is already obese or gaining weight rapidly, and are summarised in the box below. You will need more time to explore the issues in depth, and to offer an assessment that should include the child's growth, development, any unusual features or abnormalities, as well as the parent–child relationship, the home setting and any health concerns that might be linked to obesity.

Growth

Accurate growth measurements are an important part of any assessment and must be plotted onto a growth chart, making adjustment for the baby's gestational age. It takes particular skill to interpret growth patterns in the first year of life, and evaluation of obesity and rapid weight gain is no exception. One particular difficulty is interpreting weight in relation to length. In babyhood, unlike other times of life, weight is a more useful measure than Body Mass Index (BMI). Weight charts are preferable because obesity tends to drive a baby to grow in length, so calculation of BMI, which takes length into account, tends to underestimate the significance of the weight gain. However, it is still important to measure the length and head circumference.

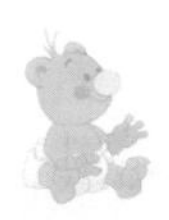

ISSUES TO EXPLORE WHEN A BABY IS AT PARTICULAR RISK FOR OBESITY

The baby/young child

- ANY concerns about the baby/young child
- Eating pattern and appetite
- Diet
- Play and activity levels
- Developmental milestones
- Behavioural problems
- Medical issues

The family

- Family history of obesity, heart disease and diabetes
- Family eating patterns and activity

Parenting

- Parenting style
- Parental attitude to food, any history of eating disorders
- Parental mental health and learning difficulties

Social and cultural context of the family

- Child care and any other influential adults
- Ethnicity and cultural/religious issues
- Involvement with social services

Beyond the age of 2 years it is valuable to calculate BMI, and you may wish to measure waist circumference as well from the age of 3 years. BMI is calculated using the formula:

$$\frac{\textit{weight (kg)}}{\textit{height (m)}^2}$$

The UK 1990 BMI charts and the UK 1990 waist circumference charts, for both girls and boys, are given in Appendix 1.

Developmental assessment and congenital or dysmorphic features

It is rare for there to be a medical cause or a syndrome underlying a child's obesity, and these are almost always identifiable on clinical assessment. The clues lie in finding delayed or disordered development, congenital abnormalities or dysmorphic features. These findings are described later in this chapter.

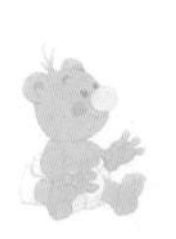

OBSERVATIONS TO INCLUDE WHEN A BABY IS AT RISK FOR OBESITY OR OBESE

Measurements

- Weight
- Length
- Head circumference
- Waist circumference from age 3

Growth chart and BMI chart

Short length or a small head may indicate a genetic or hormonal cause for excessive weight gain

Developmental progress

Developmental problems or delay may affect weight gain, eating and activity levels

Unusual features

Unusual facial features and other congenital abnormalities suggest that there might be a genetic cause for excessive weight gain

Parent–child interaction

A wealth of information can be gained by observing how the parent and child interact with each other. This can be used in helping the family understand and tackle many issues.

Home environment

Seeing the family in their home environment will also help you understand how they relate to each other, their issues, and any difficulties they may encounter in making lifestyle changes

Parent–child interaction and the home

Health practitioners are usually experienced in making the most of their informal observations of parent–child interaction and the home when seeing a family. This is a crucial part of your assessment where there are concerns about obesity. Practitioners do not often suggest that they visit at a mealtime to observe how the child eats, though parents usually welcome this if they are worried. A full discussion of how to approach and get the most out of observing a mealtime is included in Chapter 5.

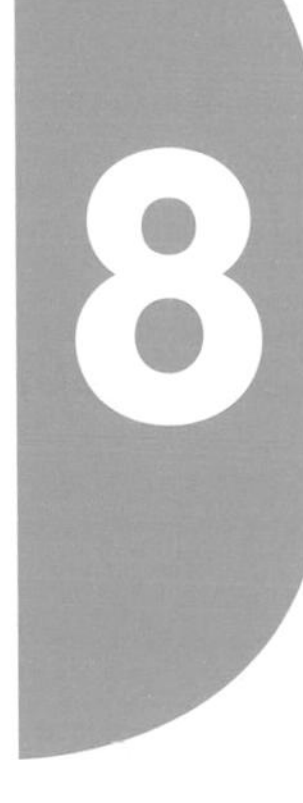

Health consequences of obesity

Preschool children are too young to develop most of the health problems that commonly occur in older individuals who are obese. They are, however, more prone to asthma, and also to sleep disturbances. Sleep apnoea (when extra fat around the upper airways blocks

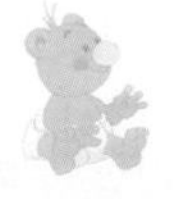

the oxygen supply to the brain at night) is of particular concern. You should suspect this if parents report snoring, gaps in the child's breathing at night and hyperactivity or lethargy during the day. You may also come across Blount's disease, where marked obesity can result in bowing of the legs.

Patterns of weight gain that are cause for concern

As described in Chapter 1, a number of studies have shown that large babies, and babies who gain weight rapidly, are more likely to be obese later in life. These studies are important as they have challenged our traditional notion that fat babies grow out of their 'podginess' and slim down in toddlerhood. Of course many will do so, but we can no longer be complacent about excessive weight gain during babyhood. It is important to be aware of this, and to share your understanding with parents, when patterns of weight gain indicate that a baby may be at increased risk. The boy's weight chart shown below illustrates some examples of weight patterns that are linked to obesity later in life.

Weight patterns indicating obesity risk

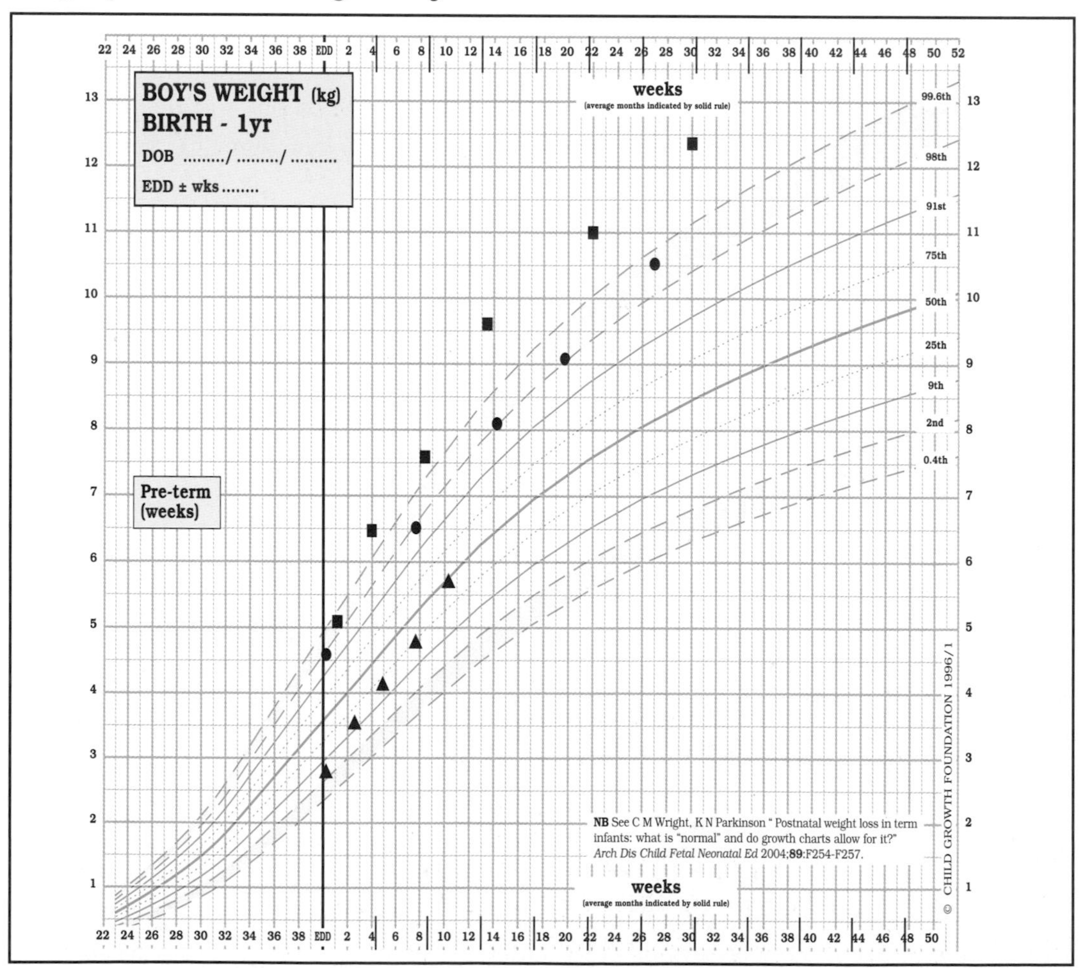

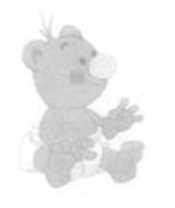

Large babies

Long-term studies clearly show that large babies are more likely to develop obesity as children and adults, but they do not give us a definite cut-off point where the risk is so high that we can predict with confidence that a baby will be obese. The chances simply increase the higher on the centiles the baby's weight lies. In the UK we tend to take the 98th weight centile as the level of concern, but that may not in practice be the cut-off we should choose. It is probably more reasonable to suggest that if a baby's weight is above the 99.6th centile, you should discuss this with the parents.

Rapid and excessive weight gain

Rapid and excessive weight gain are also predictors of later obesity, but how should we define when weight gain is rapid or excessive? This is an important question as it is common, if not usual, for babies to cross centile lines in their first year. At the present time there is no clear-cut answer to the question, but it seems reasonable to reflect in reverse the definitions we use for babies who show faltering growth or failure to thrive.

In weight faltering we generally accept that crossing two centile lines is an indication that weight gain should be monitored. So too, in rapid weight gain, crossing two centile lines in a short period of time should be an indication for assessment. This holds true even when a baby is small and demonstrating catch-up growth, as studies show that they are at higher risk of obesity as well as high blood pressure and diabetes. It has to be said that this presents some serious questions to those of us who have focused much attention on encouraging weight gain in babies who are born small. We may well need to have a major rethink about the identification and management of failure to thrive and weight faltering.

In order to help us gain a more accurate understanding of when weight gain is appropriate or not, the Child Growth Foundation has developed a practical method for practitioners to use when seeing babies for either failure to thrive or rapid weight gain. These 'thrive lines' have already been adopted by health visiting services in some parts of the country. The method involves laying an acetate sheet over the child's growth chart (in the red book or hospital notes). The lines enable you to see if weight gain over a period of 4 weeks lies outside the normal range for the child's age. If the thrive lines are crossed in an upward direction, you can be sure that the weight gain is unusually rapid.

Is measurement of length useful?

Although adjusting for length in babyhood is not helpful in defining overweight, as discussed above, it is important to measure length and head circumference. The reason for this is that both shortness in length and microcephaly in conjunction with obesity suggest that there might be a hormonal or genetic cause (see below).

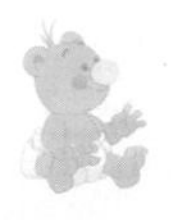

Working with families where obesity is a concern

Many health professionals feel uncomfortable about broaching the issue of obesity, when they see a baby is obese or gaining weight rapidly. This is particularly the case where parents are obese and if it is, correctly or incorrectly, assumed that they are poorly motivated to address the issue. Parents readily pick up on such attitudes – our research shows that parents who have sought help for their obese children often feel judged and that their concerns are dismissed out of hand. It is a crucial skill to be able sensitively to raise the issue of excessive weight gain, discuss concerns, help parents find their motivation and support them in making lifestyle changes.

It is often helpful to begin by considering how a healthy start is important for *all* babies. When weight gain is excessive or there is obesity in the family it simply means that it is even more important for parents to work towards establishing a healthy lifestyle in the early years. Many parents appreciate this, and if they are themselves obese they are often more determined that their children will not suffer as they have done.

It is important that we make clear, however, that although a weight pattern may be concerning, it does not mean that it is *inevitable* that the baby will become obese. It would be a great and potentially damaging disservice to label a baby in this way and generate unnecessary parental anxiety. Anxiety is damaging for both parent and baby, and the effects can be long-lasting. (For example, studies show that parents whose babies test falsely positive for a birth defect still have high anxiety levels months later, even though they know within days of the birth that there is in reality no problem.)

It would also be regrettable if, as a result of this anxiety, parents put their young children on a diet. This can not only harm the child's growth, it is also unhelpful for the development of healthy eating patterns later in life (see Chapter 5 on restrictive feeding styles). It is therefore a skill of the highest order to be able to raise the issue of concerning weight gain with parents in a way that will encourage motivation rather than provoke anxiety.

Extremely obese babies and toddlers

Severe obesity in a baby presents a number of difficulties. Parents are often aware of the social problems their child may encounter on growing up, as well as being concerned about increased health risks. They are also likely to have more immediate concerns, which may include:

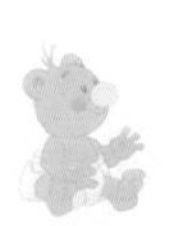

TOOLS TO USE WHEN A BABY IS AT PARTICULAR RISK OF OBESITY

BMI and waist circumference charts
These are helpful with children over 2 years to demonstrate whether the child is overweight and by how much

Thrive lines
These are useful in helping you decide if weight gain is satisfactory or excessive.

Mealtime observation (see Chapter 5)
Observing the child eat will provide you with useful information on mealtime behaviour, the parent's feeding style in particular and parenting style in general, as well as the child's diet.

Recording a mealtime (see Chapter 5)
When there are particularly difficult issues, you and the parents may find it helpful to record a mealtime and watch it together to gain a better understanding of them.

Dietary recall (see Chapter 6)
Parents can be vague about what their child eats, and it may be helpful to go over what the child eats in a structured way.

Food diary (see Chapter 6)
If you have concerns about what the child is eating, asking the parents to keep a diary for 3 days can clarify the quality and quantity of nutrients consumed. A dietitian may be needed to interpret it.

Activity diary (see Chapter 7)
This can be used as a platform for exploring activity levels and how to increase them.

Edinburgh depression scale
If there is a possibility that the mother is suffering from postnatal depression, the Edinburgh depression scale can help guide you towards suggesting professional help.

- strain when lifting and carrying their baby
- trying to control food intake in a baby who is incessantly hungry
- difficulty in buying age-appropriate clothing
- trouble in buying first shoes as the feet are too chubby
- difficulty in developing mobility because of excessive weight
- problems when shopping if the toddler is too large to sit in a supermarket trolley

In earlier chapters we have explored ways of working with parents. The more extreme the issues, the more we need to remind ourselves (and the harder this may be) that a partnership approach is likely to have good outcomes, and an expert approach likely to alienate the very parents we most need to support. In the box on page 139 you will see a summary of some of the tools we have discussed earlier in this book that may help clarify the issues and steps that might be taken. Using these within the framework of a helping relationship will encourage parents to feel supported rather than threatened.

Any baby with extreme obesity and very rapid weight gain should be offered a paediatric opinion to make sure there is not a metabolic cause or syndrome underlying the excessive weight gain. This assessment usually involves a detailed physical examination and blood tests such as thyroid function tests, chromosomes and DNA analysis.

Although it is rare that a metabolic cause is found, it is reasonable to acknowledge that obese babies may have metabolic or at least appetite differences that allow them to gain weight so excessively. Parents often find it helpful if you discuss this as a possibility, although you also need to be clear that it may well be years before we fully understand how individuals' metabolism varies. Most parents appreciate this and understand that whatever the cause of rapid weight gain, there is no alternative to lifestyle modification for tackling the problem in young children. The discussion often allows you to move on exploring together how the family's lifestyle might change. At times it is hard as some obese babies and toddlers seem to eat quite healthily and may be very active. When babies are very obese you may find it helpful to seek dietetic advice. Reducing the fat content of the diet seems sensible, so advising fat-free milk even in babyhood may be an option, though caution is needed as skimmed milk lacks some essential vitamins.

What about breast-fed babies?

Some breast-fed babies show very rapid weight gain and become quite obese. Should our concerns extend to them too? We know that breast milk has protective effects, yet it is hard to be confident in the face of such weight gain that obesity will not persist into childhood and beyond.

Until more evidence comes to light about breast-fed babies, the way is straightforward. We need to explain the limit of our understanding to parents, while reassuring them that their baby's weight is less likely to be an issue than it would be if he or she were bottle-fed. It has to be in the baby's best interests that they follow the recommendations even more closely – maintaining breastfeeding, deferring weaning until the baby is 6 months old, and providing a healthy lifestyle throughout childhood.

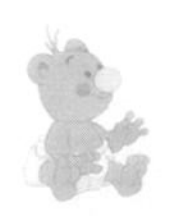

When might there be a medical or hormonal cause?

Families often believe that a genetic or metabolic problem is the cause of their child's obesity. Although there is undoubtedly a strong genetic component, a true genetic or hormonal cause is very rare. Current thinking is that about 60% of obesity is linked to genetic factors, and about 40% is environmental. It is often helpful to explain this to families, as it reduces a sense of blame or guilt.

If a baby has one of the rare syndromes that cause obesity, it is important to identify this early so that a diagnosis can be made and intensive input provided to prevent the profound obesity that can develop. Characteristics that should alert you that there might be an identifiable cause include unusual facial features and developmental delay, particularly if there are also congenital defects (see box below).

FEATURES SUGGESTING A GENETIC OR HORMONAL CAUSE FOR OBESITY

- Short stature
- Voracious insatiable appetite (hyperphagia)
- Onset of obesity before the age of 2 years
- Severe unremitting obesity
- Dysmorphic features
- Microcephaly
- Learning disability
- Hypotonia
- Hypogonadism (small genitals)
- Eye abnormalities
- Skeletal abnormalities
- Sensorineural deafness
- Renal abnormalities
- Cardiac abnormalities

The growth chart can also provide clues, as these babies commonly are short or grow poorly in length while they gain in weight. Occasionally this sort of growth pattern can be due to a hormonal cause, such as hypothyroidism, Cushing's disease or growth hormone deficiency. It is vital to identify these as they are treatable.

If any of the features in the box are present, you should ask for a paediatric opinion as investigations may be needed. If a baby is long and is developing normally, it is likely that there is no underlying medical cause for the weight gain.

Syndromes and developmental disabilities

Developmental disorders and disability need special consideration for two reasons. One is that developmental problems may point to an underlying genetic syndrome, and the other is that they may place the baby at increased risk for obesity and its complications. In both circumstances obesity prevention has an important part to play, and the early years are particularly crucial.

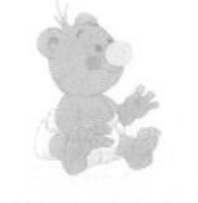

Genetic syndromes

Although genetic syndromes causing obesity are very rare, they are important as they provide us with some understanding of the metabolic abnormalities that lead to obesity. For some a single gene is responsible, and these conditions are more likely in Asian or other communities where consanguinity is common. Other syndromes have a more complex genetic cause. The metabolic pathways involved in the development of obesity are not clearly understood. It may be that the problem lies in the hypothalamus, the area of the brain responsible for appetite control. These babies and young children usually have insatiable appetites that drive their obesity.

One exceptionally rare condition is leptin deficiency. It is important to mention this as it has increased our understanding of the hormonal pathways that relate to obesity. Leptin is one of the hormones controlling appetite, and daily injections of leptin in someone who is deficient allows them to return to a normal weight in a matter of months. When first discovered, it was hoped that leptin injections might offer a solution for any obese individual, but in fact it works only for those who are leptin deficient.

The most common obesity syndrome is Prader Willi syndrome. Children born with this syndrome develop a voracious appetite that may lead to scavenging for food and massive weight gain. As babies they have poor tone and developmental delay, and boys often have small genitalia or undescended testicles. In the first year or two of life they fail to thrive, but as toddlers their appetite increases dramatically and weight gain starts. Guidance and support from a dietitian can help parents control their child's eating behaviour and therefore the obesity. The drive to eat is so powerful that parents may need to put locks on cupboard and fridge doors. Because the children have learning disabilities the situation is particularly difficult for them and for their parents.

If a genetic syndrome is identified, the baby or toddler should come under the care of a developmental paediatrician. The family should also be put in touch with the appropriate self-help organisation as these can offer valuable extra support.

Disabilities and obesity

In any individual, obesity results when there is an imbalance between nutritional intake and energy output. Disability can influence both sides of the equation. In disabilities where children's mobility is limited, weight gain is often a problem. A good example is Down's syndrome, in which the child's hypotonia leads them to be less active and their weight to rise as a result. Cerebral palsy is another example.

In these circumstances the child needs extra encouragement to be mobile, and a physiotherapist may be helpful in suggesting ways to maximise activity. Inevitably, though, adjustments are also needed in nutritional intake. As ever, prevention is easier than cure,

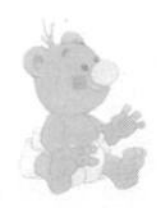

and if a baby has a condition that affects mobility it is important for parents to receive support about a lifestyle that is healthy for their child before obesity develops and becomes a concern.

When a child with a disability enters nursery or school, the focus of attention tends to be on their educational needs. Where obesity is a problem, tackling it should also be considered a special need. A great deal can be done in the structured setting that school provides, although it is usually necessary to highlight this and ensure that it is included in educational planning.

When is obesity a child protection issue?

A significant concern that has recently arisen is how obesity may relate to child abuse and neglect. This issue has caused a good deal of controversy, and will continue to do so until our understanding of obesity advances.

We still have a lot to learn about the relationship between obesity and abuse. There is certainly evidence from adult obesity clinics that some unfortunate women become obese following sexual abuse in childhood. However, it does not follow that significant numbers of children become obese because of abuse or neglect. Obesity is a complex condition, with many factors leading to weight gain. It is not appropriate to consider that obesity per se is a child protection issue, though measures must of course be considered if there are other factors in the family's history or circumstances that arouse your concern.

It may on the surface seem justifiable to condemn parents for failing to take an obese child's health seriously. If parents do not prioritise their obese child's health, surely this is an indication of neglect? However, it is clear that reversing obesity is extremely difficult. It can be a real challenge even for the best parents to control their child's weight in the face of abnormal appetite control and a social environment that is so conducive to weight gain. Parents whose lives are very troubled may not be able to give the issue the priority it needs. While we need to raise our concern and ensure that its importance is understood, we also need to accept the family's own perspective on their priorities. It is of course important that families are assured that support will still be available at a later time.

It is nevertheless possible that you may encounter a child whose immediate health or even life could be threatened. The most immediate threat is where a child develops significant airways obstruction and sleep apnoea as a result of obesity, or where complications, notably diabetes, have developed. If parents do not appear to be taking the situation seriously, child protection concerns may well need to be raised, and social services informed. It may occasionally be necessary in extreme cases to admit a child to hospital for a period, and introduce a structured eating and activity regime, along with

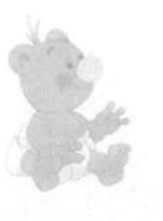

healthy lifestyle education. Weight reduction will inevitably be achieved in this artificial setting, and with ongoing support may lead to maintenance of a healthier weight following discharge. Maintaining weight reduction back at home is, however, difficult. If the situation is life-threatening child protection procedures may need to be initiated. This will always be a difficult decision, and it needs to be emphasised that this extreme action is only very rarely appropriate.

Special parental circumstances

There are a number of circumstances that may affect they way you work with parents. One that may be uncomfortable is when the parents themselves are very obese. This requires real sensitivity, and in this circumstance the HENRY approach can be particularly helpful. Parents tell us that it is not uncommon for them to feel judged by health professionals, and we need to do everything we possibly can to demonstrate a respectful attitude that will help build a positive relationship.

When trust has been established, many parents will be open to receiving help because they are unhappy with their weight and have had a difficult time coming to terms with it. Difficulties they experienced as children are likely to make them determined to prevent their child suffering in the same way, and we can help them harness this motivation. Sometimes, the desire to help their children will enable them to make changes for themselves that have not been possible before. There may, of course, be genetic tendencies in parents as well as in children that make it even harder to slow down weight gain. There is no simple answer to this; focusing on helping them achieve lifestyle change is always likely to be helpful.

Parental mental health problems present a particular difficulty. Probably the most important problem health visitors encounter is postnatal depression. A mother who is depressed will almost certainly find it difficult to be responsive to her baby; one probable result of this is that the baby will not learn to listen to their own hunger and fullness cues. They may also be in danger of being overfed as a depressed mother may respond to crying by feeding inappropriately. A vicious circle can be set up in which the mother's depression provokes anxiety in the baby, who is likely to be fretful, which the mother may try to deal with by feeding because the baby's crying worsens her depression.

Other mental health problems may also have an impact on a child's eating patterns and lifestyle. These include parental eating disorders, obsessive compulsive disorder and anxiety disorders.

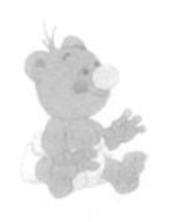

Social and cultural issues

Ethnicity has a part to play in obesity. Some ethnic groups are particularly prone to becoming obese, and more prone to develop the health problems (morbidity) that result too. This is true of the Hispanic population in the United States, and the Asian and Black communities in the UK. In general it seems that the problem particularly occurs when people from these ethnic groups are exposed to the Western diet and lifestyle. Their bodies are even less able to cope with its excesses than those of us who have lived in the West for generations.

Working with parents from different cultures also requires extra sensitivity. Lifestyle issues, and of course diet, may be different, and there may also be strong influences from the wider family. There may be different perceptions of obesity that can make the family less responsive to exploring the issues. In communities where infant mortality is traditionally high, for example, a well-fed baby would have had a greater chance of survival and overweight babies are therefore regarded as healthy.

Poverty is the other major factor that has an influence on obesity in a community. Disadvantaged children are at higher risk than their more affluent neighbours. It is undoubtedly harder to have a healthy lifestyle in circumstances where fruit and vegetables are expensive and less available, where there are fewer play spaces and it may be dangerous for a child to be out of doors without adult supervision. The solutions to these issues must be political, but in the meantime practitioners may be able to have some impact on helping families who live in disadvantaged areas.

When do you need to involve other professionals or agencies?

Working closely with other colleagues in a team environment can make the work more effective and more rewarding. Sadly, nutrition teams are not available in most parts of the country at present. Community and health practitioners need to be aware of when they need to involve colleagues, and – in discussion with families – to make referrals when appropriate. These circumstances are outlined in the box. These circumstances are outlined in the box on page 146.

REFERRALS TO BE CONSIDERED	
General practitioner	Parental mental health concerns Parental obesity (if parents wish to address this)
Child and adolescent mental health services	Behavioural concerns Severe maternal mental health concerns
Dietitian	Child's diet is very limited in variety Obesity is so extreme that restriction needs to be considered
Paediatrician/paediatric endocrinologist	Extreme obesity or very rapid weight gain before the age of 2 years Suspicion of a genetic or hormonal cause of obesity Sleep apnoea Severe bowing of the legs (Blount's disease)
Social services	Severe concerns about parenting abilities Identification of a child in need

Endword

This chapter focuses on how to help families where a baby or toddler is already obese or is gaining weight rapidly. It highlights when you should consider the possibility of a medical or genetic cause, though for most babies this will not be the case. Working to help families achieve lifestyle change is always a challenge; we have outlined family circumstances that make this all the more difficult. There is no doubt that the challenge is greater when trying to reverse obesity rather than prevent it, so early intervention is crucial. We hope that exploring the HENRY approach has encouraged you to develop a way of working that benefits both you as a practitioner and the families you support.

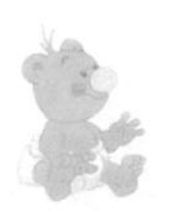

References, further reading and resources

Child Growth Foundation. BMI and waist circumference charts based on 1990 UK BMI reference curves. Designed and published by Child Growth Foundation. Supplied by Harlow Printing Ltd.

Cole TJ. 3-in-1 weight-monitoring chart. *Lancet* 1997. 349:102–3

Cox J, Holden J. *Perinatal Mental Health: A Guide to the Edinburgh Postnatal Depression Scale* The Royal College of Psychiatrists 2003

Farooqi S, O'Rahilly S. Genetics of obesity in humans *Endocrine Reviews* 2006. 27: 710–18

NHS Centre for Reviews and Dissemination. Effective health care: the prevention and treatment of childhood obesity. *NHS Centre for Reviews and Dissemination* 2002;7 (6).

Poskitt E, Edmunds L. *Management of Childhood Obesity* Cambridge University Press 2008

RCPE. Management of obesity in children and young people: a national clinical guideline. *Scottish Intercollegiate Guidelines Network* 69. April 2003. Published by Royal College of Physicians, Edinburgh. http://www.sign.ac.uk/.

RCPCH. *An approach to weight management in children and adolescents in primary care.* Produced for the Royal College of Paediatrics and Child Health and National Obesity Forum 2003.

Reilly JJ, Methven E, McDowell ZC, et al. Health consequences of obesity *Archives of Diseases in Childhood* 2003;88:748–52.

Rudolf MCJ. The obese child *Archives of Disease in Childhood Educ Pract Ed* (DVD) 2004; 89:ep57–62

Rudolf M, Hunt C. *Tuning in to Mealtimes – helping parents and carers develop responsive feeding* www.henry.org.uk

Speiser P, Rudolf MCJ et al. Consensus development: childhood obesity *Journal of Clinical Endocrinology and Metabolism* 2005. 90(3): 1871–1887

Viner R, Nicholls D. Managing obesity in secondary care: a personal practice *Archives of Disease in Childhood* 2005. 90: 385–90.

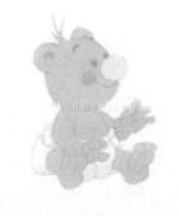

Websites

The Child Growth Foundation
www.childgrowthfoundation.org

The Prader Willi Syndrome Association
http://pwsa.co.uk

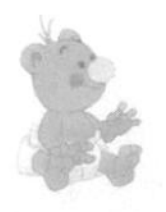

APPENDIX 1

BMI AND WAIST CIRCUMFERENCE CHARTS

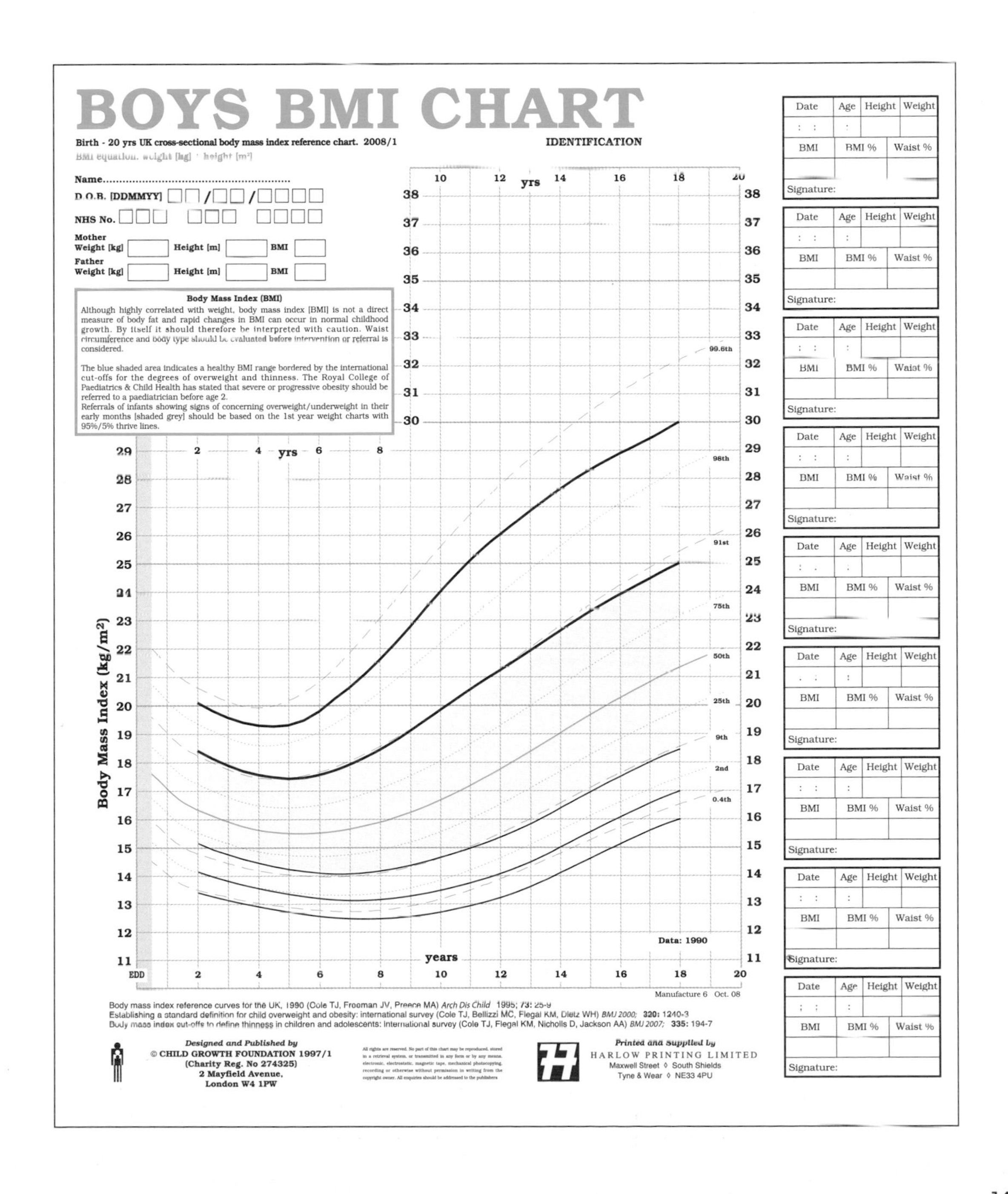

GIRLS BMI CHART

Birth - 20 yrs UK cross-sectional body mass index reference chart. 2008/1

BMI equation: weight [kg] ÷ height [m²]

IDENTIFICATION

Name...

D.O.B. [DDMMYY] ☐☐ / ☐☐ / ☐☐☐☐

NHS No. ☐☐☐ ☐☐☐ ☐☐☐☐

Mother
Weight [kg] ☐ **Height [m]** ☐ **BMI** ☐

Father
Weight [kg] ☐ **Height [m]** ☐ **BMI** ☐

Body Mass Index (BMI)

Although highly correlated with weight, body mass index [BMI] is not a direct measure of body fat and rapid changes in BMI can occur in normal childhood growth. By itself it should therefore be interpreted with caution. Waist circumference and body type should be evaluated before intervention or referral is considered.

The blue shaded area indicates a healthy BMI range bordered by the international cut-offs for the degrees of overweight and thinness. The Royal College of Paediatrics & Child Health has stated that severe or progressive obesity should be referred to a paediatrician before age 2.
Referrals of infants showing signs of concerning overweight/underweight in their early months [shaded grey] should be based on the 1st year weight charts with 95%/5% thrive lines.

Body Mass Index (kg/m²)

38 37 36 35 34 33 32 31 30 29 28 27 26 25 24 23 22 21 20 19 18 17 16 15 14 13 12 11

10 12 yrs 14 16 18 20

2 4 yrs 6 8

99.6th
98th
91st
75th
50th
25th
9th
2nd
0.4th

Data: 1990

years

EDD 2 4 6 8 10 12 14 16 18 20

Manufacture 6 Oct. 08

Body mass index reference curves for the UK, 1990 (Cole TJ, Freeman JV, Preece MA) *Arch Dis Child* 1995; **73:** 25-9

Establishing a standard definition for child overweight and obesity: international survey (Cole TJ, Bellizzi MC, Flegal KM, Dietz WH) *BMJ 2000;* **320:** 1240-3

Body mass index cut-offs to define thinness in children and adolescents: international survey (Cole TJ, Flegal KM, Nicholls D, Jackson AA) *BMJ 2007;* **335:** 194-7

Designed and Published by
© CHILD GROWTH FOUNDATION 1997/1
(Charity Reg. No 274325)
2 Mayfield Avenue,
London W4 1PW

Printed and Supplied by
HARLOW PRINTING LIMITED
Maxwell Street ◊ South Shields
Tyne & Wear ◊ NE33 4PU

Date	Age	Height	Weight
: :	:		
BMI	BMI %	Waist %	
Signature:			

Date	Age	Height	Weight
: :	:		
BMI	BMI %	Waist %	
Signature:			

Date	Age	Height	Weight
: :	:		
BMI	BMI %	Waist %	
Signature:			

Date	Age	Height	Weight
: :	:		
BMI	BMI %	Waist %	
Signature:			

Date	Age	Height	Weight
: :	:		
BMI	BMI %	Waist %	
Signature:			

Date	Age	Height	Weight
: :	:		
BMI	BMI %	Waist %	
Signature:			

Date	Age	Height	Weight
: :	:		
BMI	BMI %	Waist %	
Signature:			

Date	Age	Height	Weight
: :	:		
BMI	BMI %	Waist %	
Signature:			

Date	Age	Height	Weight
: :	:		
BMI	BMI %	Waist %	
Signature:			

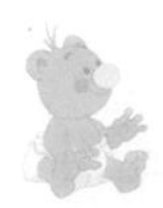

Date	Age	Height	Weight
: :	:		
BMI	BMI %	Waist %	
Signature:			

Date	Age	Height	Weight
: :	:		
BMI	BMI %	Waist %	
Signature:			

Date	Age	Height	Weight
: :	:		
BMI	BMI %	Waist %	
Signature:			

Date	Age	Height	Weight
: :	:		
BMI	BMI %	Waist %	
Signature:			

Date	Age	Height	Weight
: :	:		
BMI	BMI %	Waist %	
Signature:			

Date	Age	Height	Weight
: :	:		
BMI	BMI %	Waist %	
Signature:			

Date	Age	Height	Weight
: :	:		
BMI	BMI %	Waist %	
Signature:			

Date	Age	Height	Weight
: :	:		
BMI	BMI %	Waist %	
Signature:			

Date	Age	Height	Weight
: :	:		
BMI	BMI %	Waist %	
Signature:			

BOYS WAIST CIRCUMFERENCE

D.O.B. [DDMMYY] □□ / □□ / □□□□

Tape

Because a high BMI by itself may not be a guarantor of obesity/overweight, a high waist centile added to a high BMI centile will confirm fatness more conclusively. The shaded area represents a healthy waist range.

Measuring the Waist

The waist is defined as the mid-way point between the lowest rib cage and the iliac crest and should be measured, preferably, with a special tension tape [see illustrations below].

When measuring his waist, the boy should ideally be wearing only underclothes. Ask him to stand with his feet together and weight evenly distributed with his arms relaxed. Ask him to breathe normally and take the waist measurement at the end of a normal expiration.

The waist can also be identified by asking him to bend to one side. Measurement is taken at the point of flexure.

If he is wearing a shirt or vest, deduct 1cm before recording and plotting the waist measurement.

There is no consensus about how to define paediatric obesity using waist measurement. For clinical use the 99.6th or 98th centiles are suggested cut offs for obesity and the 91st centile for overweight, like the BMI [see chart overleaf].

years: 3 4 5 6 7 8 9 10 11 12 13 14 15 16 17

cm: 114 112 110 108 106 104 102 100 98 96 94 92 90 88 86 84 82 80 78 76 74 72 70 68 66 64 62 60 58 56 54 52 50 48 46 44 42 40

99.6th, 98th, 91st, 75th, 50th, 25th, 9th, 2nd, 0.4th

Data: 1977

Reference
The development of waist circumference percentiles in British children aged 5-16.9 yrs: (McCarthy HD et al) *European Journal of Clinical Nutrition* (2001): **55:** 902-907.

Key: % = percentile

Date	Age	Height	Weight
: :	:		
BMI	BMI %	Waist %	
Signature:			

Date	Age	Height	Weight
: :	:		
BMI	BMI %	Waist %	
Signature:			

Date	Age	Height	Weight
: :	:		
BMI	BMI %	Waist %	
Signature:			

Date	Age	Height	Weight
: :	:		
BMI	BMI %	Waist %	
Signature:			

Date	Age	Height	Weight
: :	:		
BMI	BMI %	Waist %	
Signature:			

Date	Age	Height	Weight
: :	:		
BMI	BMI %	Waist %	
Signature:			

Date	Age	Height	Weight
: :	:		
BMI	BMI %	Waist %	
Signature:			

Date	Age	Height	Weight
: :	:		
BMI	BMI %	Waist %	
Signature:			

Date	Age	Height	Weight
: :	:		
BMI	BMI %	Waist %	
Signature:			

GIRLS WAIST CIRCUMFERENCE

D.O.B. [DDMMYY] ☐☐ / ☐☐ / ☐☐☐☐

Tape

Because a high BMI by itself may not be a guarantor of obesity/overweight, a high waist centile added to a high BMI centile will confirm fatness more conclusively. The shaded area represents a healthy waist range.

Measuring the Waist

The waist is defined as the mid-way point between the lowest rib cage and the iliac crest and should be measured, preferably, with a special tension tape [see illustrations below].

When measuring her waist, the girl should ideally be wearing only underclothes. Ask her to stand with her feet together and weight evenly distributed with her arms relaxed. Ask her to breathe normally and take the waist measurement at the end of a normal expiration.

The waist can also be identified by asking her to bend to one side. Measurement is taken at the point of flexure.

If she is wearing a shirt or vest, deduct 1cm before recording and plotting the waist measurement.

There is no consensus about how to define paediatric obesity using waist measurement. For clinical use the 99.6th or 98th centiles are suggested cut-offs for obesity and the 91st centile for overweight, like the BMI [see chart overleaf].

years: 3 4 5 6 7 8 9 10 11 12 13 14 15 16 17

cm: 108 106 104 102 100 98 96 94 92 90 88 86 84 82 80 78 76 74 72 70 68 66 64 62 60 58 56 54 52 50 48 46 44 42 40 38 36 34

99.6th, 98th, 91st, 75th, 50th, 25th, 9th, 2nd, 0.4th

Data: 1977

Reference
The development of waist circumference percentiles in British children aged 5-16.9 yrs: (McCarthy HD et al) *European Journal of Clinical Nutrition* (2001): **55:** 902-907.